Handbook of the Dually Diagnosed Patient

Psychiatric and Substance Use Disorders

Handbook of the Dually Diagnosed Patient

Psychiatric and Substance Use Disorders

Sylvia J. Dennison, M.D.
Chief of Addiction Psychiatry
University of Illinois at Chicago
Chicago, Illinois

 LIPPINCOTT WILLIAMS & WILKINS
A **Wolters Kluwer** Company
Philadelphia · Baltimore · New York · London
Buenos Aires · Hong Kong · Sydney · Tokyo

Acquisitions Editor: Charles W. Mitchell
Developmental Editor: Joanne Bersin
Production Editor: Emily Lerman
Manufacturing Manager: Colin J. Warnock
Cover Designer: Patricia Gast
Compositor: Circle Graphics
Printer: R. R. Donnelley, Crawfordsville

© 2003 by LIPPINCOTT WILLIAMS & WILKINS
530 Walnut Street
Philadelphia, PA 19106 USA
LWW.com

Printed in the USA

Library of Congress Cataloging-in-Publication Data

Dennison, Sylvia J.
  Handbook of the dually diagnosed patient : psychiatric and substance use
disorders / Sylvia J. Dennison.
    p. ; cm.
  Includes bibliographical references and index.
  ISBN 0-7817-3475-4 (alk. paper)
    1. Dual diagnosis—Handbooks, manuals, etc. I. Title.
  [DNLM: 1. Diagnosis, Dual (Psychiatry) 2. Mental Disorders.
3. Substance-Related Disorders. WM 141 D411h 2003]
  RC564.68 .D466 2003
  616.86—dc21

                                                                    2002043050

Care has been taken to confirm the accuracy of the information presented and
to describe generally accepted practices. However, the author and publisher are
not responsible for errors or omissions or for any consequences from application
of the information in this book and make no warranty, expressed or implied, with
respect to the currency, completeness, or accuracy of the contents of the publication. Application of this information in a particular situation remains the professional responsibility of the practitioner.

The author and publisher have exerted every effort to ensure that drug selection
and dosage set forth in this text are in accordance with current recommendations
and practice at the time of publication. However, in view of ongoing research,
changes in government regulations, and the constant flow of information relat-
ing to drug therapy and drug reactions, the reader is urged to check the package
insert for each drug for any change in indications and dosage and for added warnings and precautions. This is particularly important when the recommended agent
is a new or infrequently employed drug.

Some drugs and medical devices presented in this publication have Food and
Drug Administration (FDA) clearance for limited use in restricted research settings. It is the responsibility of the health care provider to ascertain the FDA status of each drug or device planned for use in their clinical practice.

10 9 8 7 6 5 4 3 2 1

I would like to dedicate this book to the many patients I have been privileged to serve—
a constant source of education, and to the Hogans:
Bob, Michael, and Paul—an education of a different sort.

Contents

Preface

When I was a medical student, one of my clinical instructors told us something that meant little at the time, but much since. He told my class that if each of us would collect notes and observations on one condition, an aspect of one condition, a problem likely to be encountered in one phase of a condition, and write about it, this would be a valuable contribution to medicine. What you will find, he went on to tell us, is that much of the practical information you learn—how to approach the patient, how to really initiate, titrate, stop, or combine medications—you will learn from watching other doctors and by trial and error. Everybody thinks someone else has written everything down that's fit to write and what you'll find is that's not the case.

Of course, he was correct. On the first day of the first rotation of my junior year, I was asked by a resident to write a prescription for a patient being discharged from the hospital. I couldn't do it, as no book used in any class I had taken up to that point contained such practical information. I could rattle off the differential diagnosis for malignant hypertension, but didn't have the slightest idea as to what basic information had to be given in order for a patient to be smoothly and comfortably admitted to the hospital.

On that first day, the resident had my fellow students and me shadowing him like ducklings after their mother. He wrote orders—we took notes. He wrote prescriptions—we took notes. By the end of the day we knew the practical information, none of which had been contained in a textbook up to that time.

Once I began my psychiatric residency, again my clinical instructor was proven correct. The art that is part and parcel of psychiatric practice were not contained in a book. It could only be found by observation of others. The books didn't describe how it was done.

As a teacher working with students and house staff, I have had the privilege and responsibility to set the example, just as my instructors did for me, modeling the approach to patients. In doing so, and especially in dealing with the particularly difficult population of the psychiatric patient with substance use disorders, I have become aware of how little "practical information" there is for my students to read. Therefore, in keeping with the admonition long ago to keep notes, I've done so by creating vignettes, suggesting possible ways to approach different aspects of patient care. The *Handbook of the Dually Diagnosed Patient: Psychiatric and Substance Use Disorders* was developed from those notes.

I thank Joanne Bersin and Charles W. Mitchell of Lippincott Williams & Wilkins for their encouragement during the writing of this text. I further thank my colleague Paul W. Harris, M.D., for his review, critique, and suggestions regarding the manuscript. Finally, I thank Robert D. Hogan, Ph.D., my husband and friend, who quietly supported my work throughout this project.

Handbook of the Dually Diagnosed Patient

Psychiatric and Substance Use Disorders

1

Introduction

1. Economic burden to society caused by psychiatric and substance use disorders
   a. Increased 50% between 1985 and 1992
   b. Comorbidity costs are greater than that of all medical costs
2. Multiple social consequences of comorbidity
   a. Homelessness
   b. Increased risk of victimization
   c. Increased risk of victimizing
   d. Increased risk of neglect and abuse of children
3. Medical consequences of comorbidity
   a. Shorter life expectancy
   b. Increased risk of death by homicide and suicide
   c. Increased risk of diseases of various organ systems, depending on specific substance of abuse
4. Psychiatric consequences of comorbidity
   a. Poorer compliance with treatment
   b. Substances can mimic, induce, cause, or exacerbate illnesses
   c. Generally worsens prognosis
5. Reasons for using specific substances
   a. Multiple reasons
   b. Popular notion is that of "self-medication"
   c. Reason for initiation and for perpetuation of use can differ markedly

CASE 1-1

The patient, a young man 19 years of age, was brought to the emergency room by the police. He was found ranting and raving on a street corner, threatening passersby. He was belligerent when brought in and rapidly became frankly combative. Before the patient became unmanageable, he submitted a urine sample for toxicologic screening which, as in his previous four admissions for exacerbation of psychosis, revealed cocaine. The patient repeatedly threatened staff, the police, and other patients. He refused a physical examination, indicating that snakes were eating out his intestines and if they were touched he would die. Fearing for everyone's safety, the emergency room team administered haloperidol and lorazepam in an effort to calm the young man's agitation. The patient became rigid and diaphoretic 3 hours after admission to the emergency room. Shortly thereafter, he had a series of grand mal seizures. Despite the seizure activity, the patient's vital signs plummeted. Vigorous intravenous fluid replacement and intervention for shock were initiated, but the patient failed to respond. He was pronounced dead 56 minutes after resuscitation efforts had begun. Postmortem examination revealed peritonitis and a perforated vermiform appendix.

CASE 1-2

The patient, a female attorney 28 years of age, came to the emergency room in the company of a friend. She presented with intense feelings of self-loathing, failure, and hopelessness related to having received news that she had failed to pass her bar examination. The patient was clearly intoxicated, loud, and demanding, reeking of both old and recent alcohol ingestion. The woman's friend was clearly embarrassed by the patient's behavior and tried to calm her down, but was unable to do so. When the patient turned on her friend and gave her a brutal tongue lashing, the woman left in tears. Berating the staff as inept, the patient indicated everyone would be better off if she were gone. She further stated that she would simply leave and sleep off her drinking binge if the staff would find her a way home. A cab was arranged. The next day the patient was found dead with a blood alcohol level of 0.300 and an empty bottle of diazepam on the floor beside her.

These descriptions are composites of cases—scenarios that can play out in a variety of ways in dealing with the dually diagnosed. It is easy to become focused on one aspect of the patient—the addicted part—and forget that other problems might coexist. We do not neglect to treat the hypertension in the diabetic, but we may forget that the individual with depression, a recent significant loss, and acutely under the influence of alcohol is among the highest risk for suicide of all patients. A violent young man with schizophrenia and cocaine in him can still develop an acute abdomen, neuroleptic malignant syndrome, or another life-threatening problem. Comorbidity is the rule, not the exception, when it comes to treating mentally ill patients, and the cost of comorbidity is substantial, both monetarily and otherwise.

The National Institute on Drug Abuse and the National Institute on Alcohol Abuse and Alcoholism estimate that abuse of alcohol and other drugs cost the United States $245.7 billion in 1992, the last year for which information is available. This represents a 50% increase over the cost in 1985 and includes that of treating drug-related diseases (e.g., human immunodeficiency virus), lost wages and productivity caused by absenteeism and premature death, incarceration of substance sellers and users, and crime prevention and interdiction (1).

Likewise, difficulties associated with mental illnesses place a tremendous burden on economies worldwide. A study published by the National Institute of Mental Health ranks the economic impact of all medical and psychiatric diseases on society, finding that the economic burden exerted by all mental illnesses, not including alcohol and other drug use, ranks second only to that of cardiovascular conditions. Adding substance use disorders to all other mental illnesses places the economic cost of all psychiatric conditions well ahead of all physical disorders.

Data also indicate that substance use disorders and other psychiatric conditions occur simultaneously at a high rate. Regier et al. (2) found, in a community sample, that individuals with a mental disorder had an odds ratio of 2.7 and a lifetime prevalence rate of 29% for having some addictive disorder. In treatment and institutional settings, the odds of comorbidity are even higher. Given the high cost of mental illnesses and substance use disorders to society, it is easy to see that when such conditions occur simultaneously, the economic impact will be substantial. In fact, treatment of comorbid conditions claims a disproportionate amount of the healthcare dollar. Despite recognition of the high cost of comorbidity and it prevalence, surprisingly little attention has been given to this problem until the last decade.

PROBLEMS OF SUBSTANCE ABUSE AND COMORBIDITY

Apart from the economic burden, what makes substance abuse in general, and comorbidity in particular, a problem? Primarily, social and health issues that affect both the abuser and society in general, which are briefly discussed.

Social Sequelae

Substance misuse among mentally ill individuals is associated with a lower likelihood of employment and an increased risk of poverty (3,4). This, in turn, leads to an increased risk of homelessness and homelessness is associated with an overall poorer prognosis for the mentally ill (5). The homeless mentally ill person who abuses or misuses substances is less likely to be compliant with medication and more likely to require rehospitalization for exacerbation of mental illness and be incarcerated than are mentally ill individuals who do not exhibit comorbid problems (6).

The mentally ill substance abuser is at an increased risk of being the victim of rape and other violent assault (7–12). Victimization, in turn, predicts a worsening of symptoms (13). Further, the dually diagnosed individual is at risk of being the perpetrator of such crimes as well. Although most violent crimes are not committed by the mentally ill, studies show that those that are, are disproportionately committed by those with comorbid substance use disorders. This risk of violence and victimization do not appear to be the result of criminal activity to obtain or use drugs, but of the disinhibiting effects of the substances themselves. In addition, substance use contributes to a substantial percentage of both accidental and of homicidal deaths in this population (14–18).

The user is not the only one who suffers from the social effects of substance use. Children are at increased risk of neglect and abuse by substance-using parents (19,20). In addition, a heightened risk exists of substance misuse among the children of parents who abuse substances, a fact that appears to have both environmental and genetic influences (21–23).

Physical Health

That the use of psychoactive substances is associated with a wide variety of physical ailments is well recognized. Nicotine use causes emphysema, hypertension, and various types of cancers. Heavy alcohol consumption causes problems in virtually every organ system in the human body, with particular impact on gastrointestinal, especially hepatic, functioning; blood dyscrasias; it damages the peripheral and central nervous system; and causes cardiovascular disease. Cocaine can cause hypertensive crises, stroke, ischemia in any part of the body, and myocardial infarction. The intravenous

Table 1-1.   Problems associated with comorbidity

Social
  Homelessness
  Victimization
  Incarceration
  Victimizing
  Abuse and neglect of children (if parents)
Medical
  Damage in every organ system
  Risk of infectious disease
  Disproportionate use of
    healthcare dollar
  Potential for medication: drug interaction
  Premature death from variety of causes
Mental health
  Poor medication compliance
  Rehospitalization
  Mimic, induce, cause, worsen mental illnesses
  Increased dropout rate from treatment
  Generally worsens prognosis

administration of drugs increases the risks of endocarditis, hepatitis, a host of other infectious diseases, and renal disease. This list is only a partial accounting of the physical sequelae of substance use and misuse.

Mental Health and Treatment Issues

Substances of abuse can mimic, induce, cause, or exacerbate, mental illnesses. For example, alcohol and cocaine use causes and is a consequence of depression (24,25). Both can also result in, or significantly worsen, psychoses and anxiety reactions (26–28). The use of such substances is associated with an increased risk of hospitalization among those with concomitant mental illnesses. Individuals with substance use disorders are less compliant with medication and more likely to drop out of treatment. Comorbidity, in short, is associated with a worsened prognosis overall (29,30).

Thus, although substance misuse *per se* is a source of significant social and medical morbidity, in the case of the mentally ill person, the problems become magnified many times over (Table 1-1).

WHY DO PEOPLE USE THE DRUGS THEY DO?

Why people use drugs is a question that has been asked for many years. People give a variety of reasons for using the drugs they do: to feel different, to fit in, curiosity, as a social lubricant, to avoid withdrawal symptoms, it's enjoyable; they feel better when they use it and feel bad when they do not use it. Perhaps the most popular idea and one that appeals to many in the mental health field is that of the "self-medication theory" of addictive disorders. This theory suggests that people use the substances to treat their psychological needs pharmacologically; they chemically treat something that they lack or replace something they are missing, much as a serotonin reuptake inhibiting antidepressant pushes the central nervous system to make more serotonin available in the brain. Although, typically, they try a variety of different drugs, most individuals who become physically dependent on a drug eventually gravitate to a single drug as the preferred substance of choice (31–33). For most people, however, the drugs they gravitate toward will be nicotine and alcohol, the only legal drugs. Because most people with and without psychiatric problems try to stay within the law, it is difficult to test the self-medication theory (2,34,35).

Aside from the legal aspects of the problem, there is both support and rebuttal of the theory. As noted, substance use disorders and psychiatric disorders co-occur at a high rate, consistent with the concept that those who misuse substances are "medicating " themselves. Yet, many who misuse substances do not have another diagnosis. They are simply physiologically dependent on a substance. What is their excuse under this concept?

Nay-sayers look at the fact that cocaine use is widespread among individuals with schizophrenia. Use of the drug is associated with an increase in the number of hospitalizations and a worsening of the positive symptoms of schizophrenia, hardly support for the idea that the individual is self-medicating (29,36). Supporting the concept is the finding that those same individuals with schizophrenia demonstrate improvement in the negative symptoms of their disease when they use this drug (37–40).

Unfortunately, the reason people start using a substance and the reason they continue may differ dramatically. At some point, the substance takes on a character of its own, and the individual may feel compelled to continue its use. Drugs cause changes in the nervous system that make its use self-perpetuating and take much of the volitional aspect out of the equation. This is what makes treating substance use disorders difficult: the individual feels "out of control." When a psychiatric disorder, especially a psychotic disorder, is superimposed on a substance use disorder, the problem is compounded more than doubly.

TREATING THE PATIENT WITH BOTH A PSYCHIATRIC AND A SUBSTANCE USE DISORDER

The "Dually Diagnosed"

Substance misuse in the presence of an ongoing psychiatric illness complicates treatment of both disorders. Treatment providers often feel knowledgeable about one or the other problem, but not both.

Caregivers hesitate to prescribe necessary pharmaceuticals because they fear an interaction between psychiatric medications and psychoactive substances the patient may be abusing.

Patients themselves may believe they should stop their medications if they are using alcohol and other street substances, thus exacerbating their illnesses. Because substances of abuse can cause reactions that mimic psychiatric conditions, treatment providers may fail to recognize the correct diagnosis and treat the wrong problem.

Clearly, treating the dually diagnosed patient presents the caregiver with a unique set of challenges, which, although difficult, are

Table 1-2.   Reasons for using substances of abuse

Biological	Social
Self-medication	Feels good
Substance causes changes in nervous system so individual *must* use	To feel different
Avoid withdrawal	To fit in
	"Social lubricant"
	Curiosity

not insurmountable. The following chapters discuss the increasing knowledge available about, and a decade worth of personal experience in working with, this population (Table 1-2).

REFERENCES

1. Abuse NIoD. Drug abuse cost to society set at $97.7 billion. Rockville, MD: National Institutes of Health, 1998;1:12–13.
2. Regier DA, Farmer ME, Rae DS, et al. Comorbidity of mental disorders with alcohol and other drug abuse: results from the Epidemiological Catchment Area study. *JAMA* 1990;264(19):2511–2518.
3. Mueser KT, Becker DR, Torrey WC, et al. Work and nonvocational domains of functioning in persons with severe mental illness: a longitudinal analysis. *J Nerv Ment Dis* 1997;185(7):419–426.
4. Zlotnick C, Robertson MJ, Tam T. Substance use and labor force participation among homeless adults. *Am J Drug Alcohol Abuse* 2002;28(1):37–53.
5. Sullivan G, Burnam A, Koegel P. Pathways to homelessness among the mentally ill. *Soc Psychiatry Psychiatr Epidemiol* 2000; 35(10):444–450.
6. Lamb HR, Weinberger LE. Persons with severe mental illness in jails and prisons: a review. *Psychiatr Serv* 1998;49(4):483–492.
7. Wenzel SL, Koegel P, Gelberg L. Antecedents of physical and sexual victimization among homeless women: a comparison to homeless men. *Am J Community Psychol* 2000;28(3):367–390.
8. Goldfinger SM, Schutt RK, Turner W, et al. Assessing homeless mentally ill persons for permanent housing: screening for safety. *Community Ment Health J* 1996;32(3):275–288.
9. Goodman LA, Dutton MA, Harris M. Episodically homeless women with serious mental illness: prevalence of physical and sexual assault. *Am J Orthopsychiatry* 1995;65(4):468–478.
10. North CS, Smith EM, Spitznagel EL. Violence and the homeless: an epidemiologic study of victimization and aggression. *J Trauma Stress* 1994;7(1):95–110.
11. Padgett DK, Struening EL. Victimization and traumatic injuries among the homeless: Associations with alcohol, drug, and mental problems. *Am J Orthopsychiatry* 1992;62(4):525–534.
12. Zapf PA, Roesch R, Hart SD. An examination of the relationship of homelessness to mental disorder, criminal behavior, and health care in a pretrial jail population. *Can J Psychiatry* 1997; 41(7):435–440.

13. Goodman LA, Dutton MA, Harris M. The relationship between violence dimensions and symptom severity among homeless, mentally ill women. *J Trauma Stress* 1997;10(1):51–70.
14. Modestin J, Ammann R. Mental disorders and criminal behavior. *Br J Psychiatry* 1995;166(5):667–675.
15. Modestin J, Berger A, Ammann R. Mental disorder and criminality: male alcoholism. *J Nerv Ment Dis* 1996;184(7):393–402.
16. Monahan J. The prediction of violent behavior: toward a second generation of theory and practice. *Am J Psychiatry* 1984;141(1): 10–15.
17. Beaudoin MN, Hodgins S, Lavoie F. Homicide, schizophrenia and substance abuse or dependency. *Can J Psychiatry* 1993;38(8): 541–546.
18. Rasanen P, Tiihonen J, Isohanni M, et al. Schizophrenia, alcohol abuse, and violent behavior: a 26-year follow up study of an unselected birth cohort. *Schizophr Bull* 1998;24(3):437–441.
19. Dunn MG, Mezzich A, Janiszewski S, et al. Transmission of neglect in substance abuse families: the role of child dysregulation and parental SUD. *Journal of Child & Adolescent Substance Abuse* 2001;10(4):123–132.
20. Nair P, Black MM, Schuler M, et al. Risk factors for disruption in primary care-giving among infants of substance abusing women. *Child Abuse Negl* 1997;21(11):1039–1051.
21. Kosten TR, Rounsaville BJ, Kleber HD. Parental alcoholism in opioid addicts. *J Nerv Ment Dis* 1985;173(8):461–469.
22. Evans S, Levin FR, Fischman MW. Increased sensitivity to alprazolam in females with a paternal history of alcoholism. *Psychopharmacology* 2000;150(2):150–162.
23. Weitzman EA, Wechsler H. Alcohol use, abuse and related problems among children of problem drinkers: findings from a national survey of college alcohol use. *J Nerv Ment Dis* 2000;188(3): 148–154.
24. Grant BF, Harford TC. Comorbidity between DSM-IV alcohol use disorders and major depression: results of a national survey. *Drug Alcohol Depend* 1995;39(3):197–206.
25. Abraham HD, Fava M. Order of onset of substance abuse and depression in a sample of depressed outpatients. *Compr Psychiatry* 1999;40(1):44–50.
26. Rosen MI, Kosten TR. Cocaine associated panic attacks in methadone maintained patients. *Am J Drug Alcohol Abuse* 1992; 18(1):57–62.
27. Seibyl JP, Satel SL, Anthony D, et al. Effects of cocaine on hospital course in schizophrenia. *J Nerv Ment Dis* 1993;181:31–37.
28. Sevy S, Kay SR, Opler LA, et al. Significance of cocaine history in schizophrenia. *J Nerv Ment Dis* 1990;178:642–648.
29. Havassy BE, Arns PG. Relationship of cocaine and other substance dependence to well-being of high-risk psychiatric patients. *Psychiatric Serv* 1998;49(7):935–940.
30. Sonne SC, Brady KT, Morton WA. Substance abuse and bipolar affective disorder. *J Nerv Ment Dis* 1994;182(6):349–352.
31. Khantzian EJ. Self-regulation and self-medication factors in alcoholism and the addictions: similarities and differences. *Recent Dev Alcohol* 1990;8:255–271.
32. Khantzian EJ. The self-medication hypothesis of addictive disorders: focus on heroin and cocaine dependence. *Am J Psychiatry* 1985;142(11):1259–1264.

33. Wiess RD, Mirin SM. Substance abuse as an attempt at self-medication. *Psychiatric Med* 1987;3:357–367.
34. Breslau N, Kilbey MM, Andreski P. Nicotine dependence and major depression: new evidence from a prospective investigation. *Arch Gen Psychiatry* 1993;50(1):31–35.
35. Grant BF, Harford TC, Dawson DA. Prevalence of DSM-IV alcohol abuse and dependence: United States, 1992. *Alcohol Health and Research World* 1994;18(3):243–248.
36. Wolpe PR, Gorton G, Serota R, et al. Predicting compliance of dual diagnosis inpatients with aftercare treatment. *Hospital and Community Psychiatry* 1993;44(1):45–49.
37. Serper MR, Alpert M, Richardson NA, et al. Clinical effects of recent cocaine use on patients with acute schizophrenia. *Am J Psychiatry* 1995;152(10):1464–1469.
38. Lysaker P, Bell M, Goulet JB, et al. Relationship of positive and negative symptoms to cocaine abuse in schizophrenia. *J Nerv Ment Dis* 1994;182(2):109–112.
39. LeDuc PA, Mittleman G. Schizophrenia and psychostimulant abuse: a review and reanalysis of clinical evidence. *Psychopharmacology* 1995;121:407–427.
40. Dixon L, Haas G, Weiden PJ, et al. Drug abuse in schizophrenic patients: clinical correlates and reasons for use. *Am J Psychiatry* 1991;148(2):224–230.

2

The Language of Treatment and Treatment Modalities

1. Difficulties in treatment of the dually diagnosed
   a. Mental healthcare programs and addiction treatment programs ill equipped to deal with both problems
   b. Three models of care for this population, each with its own problems
   c. Best suited is integrated offering of care: few treatment programs equipped to deal with both
2. Treatment providers in addiction treatment and in mental health treatment programs do not speak the same language
   a. Enabling *vs.* assisting
   b. Drugs *vs.* medication
   c. Powerlessness *vs.* empowerment
   d. Individualization *vs.* an "addict is an addict"
3. Models of treatment
   a. Brief intervention
   b. Twelve-step self-help groups
   c. Network therapy
   d. Therapeutic community
   e. Harm reduction
   f. Methadone maintenance therapy
   g. Relapse prevention

How to treat patients suffering with both mental illnesses and substance use disorders remains a controversial issue. Researchers have been rigorously addressing this issue for less than a decade, so good data demonstrating the superiority of one approach over another are only now accumulating. Over the years, practitioners have proposed treating such patients using the following models.

1. Sequentially: two different sets of practitioners treating one problem first, then the other
2. In parallel: two different sets of treatment providers treating each problem in separate programs but at the same time
3. In integrated programs: one set of staff addressing both problems

Each of these models has its own peculiar problems. Individuals with mental health backgrounds and those coming from traditional addiction treatment orientations can have markedly different treatment philosophies. Patients treated in sequential or parallel programs often receive conflicting messages, which decreases the likelihood of a positive outcome (1,2). Integrated programs, on the other hand, suffer from a dearth of care providers truly knowledgeable about the treatment of both substance misuse and mental illness (Table 2-1).

Another problem facing the dually diagnosed patient is the widespread acceptance of 12-step self-help groups as a primary form of addiction treatment. Such programs consist of individuals who

Table 2-1.   Treatment models

Model	How It Works	Problems
Sequential	One problem treated first, followed by the other	Which to treat first Ignores impact and interaction of disorders on each other
Parallel	Problems treated simultaneously	Conflicting messages Potential for conflicting goals of programs (e.g., medication compliance *vs.* completely drug-free)
Integrated	Problems treated within same problem	Dearth of treatment providers truly knowledgeable about treatment of substance mis-use and mental illnesses

have combated their own substance use problems and often do not have trained professionals, a necessary part of mental health treatment. Dually diagnosed clients have often done poorly in tra-ditional 12-step programs, where psychiatric symptoms can be attributed solely to the substance use (3). Strict psychiatric pro-grams have not been without their problems either, however, often ignoring or misdiagnosing the addictive disorder.

Clearly, successful treatment of this difficult population re-quires that the treatment provider understand the issues facing individuals with addictive disorders and those with other men-tal disorders. They also need to know how the symptoms of each condition mimics and overlaps that of the other, and how the treatment needs of each can interact with and complicate the other (4–7). For treatment providers to acquire this understand-ing, it is necessary to develop a language understood by both men-tal health and substance abuse treatment providers. Although seemingly a simple task, such an undertaking is difficult because of the differing orientations of the two types of caregivers. Dis-cussed below are some of the conflicting perceptions of these two disparate camps (Table 2-2).

ENABLING *VS.* ASSISTING

Traditional substance abuse treatment programs insist on the individual being "ready to quit" as a criterion for admission into treatment. It is up to the individual to be motivated to change and to take responsibility for getting personal needs met. The coun-selor who attempts to take on this role is said to be "enabling" the patient.

Mental healthcare workers often see their clientele as disorga-nized and paralyzed, unable to get the help they need without much direction and support. They see their role as guiding clients through the system as "assisting" the mentally ill client, and view the substance treatment providers as uncaring.

Table 2-2.   Language differences: addiction treatment *vs.* mental health

Traditional Addiction Treatment	Mental Health
Enabling: individual must be motivated for treatment and accept responsibility for getting needs met	**Assisting:** individual with psychiatric problems is disorganized and in need of much guidance to get needs met
Drugs: abstinence from all psychoactive substances is a requirement of treatment	**Medication:** compliance with prescribed medications is a goal of treatment
Powerlessness: individual is powerless over addiction and must accept this fact to get better	**Empowerment:** individual does not have to be a victim of the disease; each person can learn to recognize signs of worsening and exert some control over them
An addict is an addict: go to meetings, read the "Big Book," and practice the teaching of AA and you'll get better	**Individualization of treatment:** people are unique and each one's problems must be approached individually and in a way designed uniquely for that person

MEDICATION *VS.* DRUGS

Often, individuals taking any psychoactive drugs, including medication, are excluded from addiction treatment programs. The rationale is that such individuals are not truly "drug-free" and should not be permitted into abstinence-only programs.

Mental health providers are careful to differentiate between "drugs" and "medications." Drugs are bought on the street. A physician prescribes medications for a mental condition and taking that medication, as prescribed, is often a treatment goal.

Mental health providers often fail to recognize the presence of a substance use disorder. Even when such is recognized, it is not uncommon for addicted individuals to be treated with addictive agents without consideration of their addiction potential, raising the ire of addiction treatment staff. This sets up a situation between the two camps in which the mental healthcare professional believes the addiction treatment provider is attempting to subvert the recommended treatment approach. The addiction treatment provider, on the other hand, may view the mental healthcare provider as naïve and uninformed, promoting addictive behaviors and possibly setting up the addicted individual for relapse.

ABSTINENCE *VS.* HARM REDUCTION

One area in which both addiction treatment and mental healthcare providers are in agreement is the only acceptable goal of treatment is that the patient must to stop using all nonprescribed psychoactive substances. Individuals testing positive for substances of abuse are often evicted from both the mental health clinic and the addiction treatment clinic simultaneously, although, of course, this is exactly the time when the individual needs help the most. A schizophrenic patient who requires hospitalization for psychosis after an alcohol binge seems to prove that alcohol use results in psychosis. Largely contributing to the psychotic process is the fact that the clinic refuses to give the patient the medication if the patient is drinking, although this fact is often overlooked.

The term "harm reduction" is relatively new on the treatment scene, although the concept has been used for several decades in the form of methadone maintenance clinics. It means exactly what it says: reduce the harm that using psychoactive substances is doing to both the user and those around that person. This approach, which is discussed in more detail later in this chapter, has not been wholeheartedly accepted by either the mental health or the addiction treatment community, although it is gaining ground in mainstream treatment programs.

POWERLESSNESS VS. EMPOWERMENT

The model of substance dependence treatment in the United States has traditionally been along the lines of Alcoholics Anonymous (AA), in which each person with a substance use problem must accept being "powerless" over addiction as a criterion for getting better. The person is told that once he or she begins to use a substance of choice, that person will inevitably lose all control and be unable to stop drug use. The mental healthcare provider attempts to help the client to be less of a "victim" of the disease. Rather than having bipolar illness and doomed to recurrent exacerbations of the mental illness, the patient is encouraged to recognize cues to worsening of his or her condition and to develop strategies for dealing with such as they occur. The intent is to empower the individual to take control of the disease to the degree possible.

INDIVIDUALIZATION OF TREATMENT
VS. AN ADDICT IS AN ADDICT

Throughout the 1970s and 1980s, addicted patients were lock-stepped into programs of the same length, with the same emphases and the same content. Individual needs were largely ignored. The justification was that "an addict is an addict." Managed care and a lack of evidence that prolonged inpatient stays improved outcome forced care providers to look at outcome, demonstrate efficacy, and provide individualized care to each patient.

Mental healthcare providers have long recognized that individuals manifest the same illness in different ways. They were used to approaching each of their clients as a unique individual, having similar illnesses, but with their own peculiar expression.

TREATMENT OF COMORBID DISORDERS

Once a common language is adopted, it is necessary for the treatment provider to decide on a treatment strategy or strategies for approaching a particular addicted individual with comorbid psychiatric difficulties. Following is a brief review of some of the interventions that have been devised for dealing with addictive disorders. It is not intended as an exhaustive review of the field.

Such is beyond the scope of this book. Rather, it is an effort to familiarize the reader with a few of the approaches that have been used in the field of addiction treatment. In addition, the reader will note that no mention is made of such psychotherapeutic approaches as cognitive behavioral therapy or psychodrama, both of which are valuable tools in the armamentarium of the therapist in the addiction field. The reason for this is that the primary focus of this book is on pharmacologic interventions. This is not an attempt to deny the importance of many of the valuable psychotherapies that exist to help the addicted or otherwise psychiatrically impaired individual. Rather, it is the possible interaction of substances of abuse with psychiatric medications that is often most problematic to the treatment provider, and not an issue that has yet received much attention. Many available texts deal with specific psychotherapeutic techniques and their application in the field of addictive disorders. The reader would do well to refer to one of these for this specific subject (Table 2-3).

BRIEF INTERVENTION

Brief intervention is an approach recommended for primary care providers to take with patients who are early in their problematic use of psychoactive substances. It consists of providing factual information regarding personal risks and recommended levels of usage (if such exist), and recommending corrective action.

CASE 2-1

David L. is a successful businessman 35 years of age. For many years, as was a tradition in his family, he has walked to the corner tavern for lunch, which consists of a sandwich and a couple of beers. Evenings, he has a couple more beers while he watches the news, wine with dinner, and a nightcap. He has no physical problems, does not drink and drive, and his wife is not concerned about his usage.

David L. is far exceeding the recommended safe level of alcohol consumption. Yet, he is not demonstrating any functional or significant physical impairment, does not need to be in a treatment program, nor does any reason exist for him to refrain from all alcohol. He should, however, be made aware of the health risks and what the safe recommended level of alcohol consumption is (no more than two standard drinks per day for men; one standard drink per day for women). In addition, he should be given some recommendations on how to modify his drinking.

12-STEP, SELF-HELP GROUPS

A common and readily available option for receiving help for addictive disorders is that of 12-step, self-help groups (e.g., Alcoholics Anonymous, Narcotics Anonymous [NA], and Cocaine Anonymous [CA]). The only requirement for membership in 12-step groups is a "sincere desire to stop" using (e.g., alcohol, drugs). The exact number of members and the efficacy rates of such groups are unknown because of the lack of empiric data and the anonymous nature of the organization. Nevertheless, assistance

Table 2-3.   Treatment approaches

Technique	Application
Brief intervention	Educational approach typically by a primary care practitioner toward a patient who is using a substance in a abusive fashion but has not yet developed significant health, social, or occupational problems as a result of it.
12-step	Individuals in recovery helping others to achieve the same. Available worldwide. No cost.
Network therapy	Uses family, friends, others to help the individual develop and practice. Keeps individual in own environment, facing real-life situations.
Therapeutic community	Individual resides in a "community" with others in various stages of recovery, typically, from heroin addiction. Anticipated length of stay a minimum of 18 months. Decisions made for the individual early on. Progresses in recovery and learns new ways of dealing with life in a drug-free fashion, which earns the individual more freedoms.
Harm reduction	Seeks to help individual minimize the damage substance use is doing to self and others. Teaches moderation rather than abstinence in most cases.
Methadone maintenance	A form of harm reduction. Supplies the individual with a long-acting opiate daily so not to risk withdrawal symptoms. Theory is that addicts are supplying themselves with something needed in the form of the opiate. The methadone clinic will supply it instead.
Relapse prevention	An approach after abstinence has been achieved, teaching the individual to develop strategies for avoiding situations that place the self at high risk of resuming patterns of using substance again and how to deal with those situations and actual relapses if they occur.

from 12-step groups is available in countries throughout the world and requires no membership fee.

The 12 steps refers to a dozen issues the individual must work through to achieve recovery from an addictive disorder. Twelve-step programs consist of individuals recovering from addictions helping others who likewise wish to achieve this goal.

Alcoholics Anonymous was the first 12-step program. Its principles have since been adopted and modified for helping heroin addicts (NA), cocaine addicts (CA), compulsive overeaters (Overeaters Anonymous [OA]), and a host of other similar organizations, collectively referred to as "self-help" groups. It was begun in the 1930s largely through the work of two men, both of whom had tried unsuccessfully on their own to overcome their difficulties with alcoholism. They believed that alcoholics like themselves would be the only people able to help other alcoholics—not doctors, not ministers, not shamans, not spiritualists, but alcoholics who knew the problem firsthand and could help each other. The acceptance of their approach is attested to by the existence of AA in many countries worldwide and meetings in a wide variety of languages. Part of the advantage of AA and similar groups is that it takes the substance user out of the using environment, away from using people, and places that person in a milieu where using is frowned on with a group of people who, similarly, are attempting to stop using.

A degree of spiritualism is associated with some 12-step groups that is not acceptable to all individuals seeking help. This is found in the form of an admonition that a "higher power" is necessary in order to recover from an addictive disorder. Programs, such as Rational Recovery, have evolved along the lines of AA, but on the premise that individuals trying to overcome addiction can do so with the help of others with similar difficulties, but that a spiritual being is not necessary for recovery.

Twelve-step groups encourage their members to attend meetings daily for support. A strong emphasis is placed on addictive disorders being life-long problems and that members will need AA for the rest of their lives.

Previously, some bias from 12-step organizations existed toward any type of medication intervention for psychiatric disorders, sometimes to the detriment of the individual seeking help. Increasingly, however, members of such organizations have become more aware of the unique needs of its members. It is now not uncommon for members to encourage one another to turn to their physicians for medication issues and to each other for help staying clean and sober.

Many, if not most, traditional addiction treatment programs require attendance at some 12-step meetings as part of the contract of receiving treatment. As noted, this may not be a good idea when dealing with a dually diagnosed patient. A movement has developed geared specifically toward this population, called "Dual Recovery" groups. The clinician is best advised to be familiar with the particular character of a given group before recommending it to, for example, a psychotic patient, who may not be ready for the emotions that can be evoked in some meetings.

If the clinician does recommend attendance at a 12-step meeting, it is a useful idea, if a variety exists, to recommend attendance at several different meetings before accepting the patient's claim that "AA isn't for me." In large cities with diverse populations, 12-step groups can take on strong personal identities. Patients who find themselves in a group with an identity radically different may not feel the level of support for sobriety that would be optimal (e.g., a person who is gay and white in a group comprised of predominately heterosexual, African–American men). It does not mean the group could not help him. It simply means he might not be able to engage as quickly as if he found himself in a group of men and women like himself or of a more diverse nature. In small rural communities, 12-step meetings may be few and far between, so choosing may not be an option.

NETWORK THERAPY

Another approach to substance misuse is that of network therapy, developed and described in detail by Galanter (8). Typically, under the supervision of a mental healthcare worker, network therapy focuses on individuals and their personal "network" of support. Persons important in the patient's life (e.g., friends, family, coworkers, employer) are recruited to assist the therapist and the addicted patient in developing and executing a plan of recovery. It uses peer pressure to help the individual remain abstinent and encourages that person to use personal social milieu to obtain the support needed for this purpose. The addicted individual is confronted by the peer group about substance use and, with the group, develops a plan for corrective action. The group reviews the individual's progress and makes changes in the plan as indicated by the person's success or failure, which keeps that person in the real world where temptations and problems exist. The purpose is to help the individual learn to cope with life without substance of abuse in a real-life setting with real-life problems and real-life support systems.

THERAPEUTIC COMMUNITY

A therapeutic community, an approach that originated in the 1950s, gained increased acceptance in the 1960s and 1970s. It has decreased in popularity because of cost and question of efficacy. This is a treatment, typically for heroin addicts, in which professional involvement is at a minimum and "therapy" consists of addicts helping other addicts learn how to live in a new, drug-free fashion. With this approach, addicted members of a household, the "community," and individuals in recovery live together in a drug-free environment. Initially, the newly abstinent addict has no freedoms or choices. The addict resides in the household with no or minimal interaction with the outside world and earns increasing privileges by maintaining a drug-free lifestyle, demonstrating mature behavior, following house rules, and participating in groups. Important decisions are made for that person. By working his or her way up the recovery ladder, and demonstrating mature, non-manipulative behaviors, the patient is permitted an increasing amount of autonomy.

CASE 2-2

At 28 years of age, Bill T. had been in and out of jail too many times to count and in prison once for robbery. He started injecting heroin at 16 years of age. His only serious periods of "clean"

*time were when he was behind bars. Now on parole, he knows he
would like to use again, but he also knows that he never wants to
be back in jail. He decided on a therapeutic community.*

*First, they shaved his head because he needed to develop some-
thing in himself to be proud of, not something on his outside, he
was told. After he tried to ingratiate himself to the psychologist
who came twice a week to lead group therapy, the house made
him carry around a can of 10-W-30 motor oil for a week to
remind him of how greasy he was.*

*At first, he got all the lousy jobs—toilet detail, dirty dishes,
scrubbing the floors—and he complained bitterly. All Bill wanted
to do was get high. Over time, however, he was too tired to care.
He stopped complaining and got the work done. He saw the new
guys come in and do a poor job and complain about it, and he was
impatient with them. More needed to be done and they needed to
do it. Sometimes, he would pitch in and help, because he did not
like to see things done poorly. At this point, Bill was graduated to
more responsibility and more freedom.*

To be successful, it is anticipated that the individual will remain
in the therapeutic community for a minimum of 18 months. Pro-
ponents of this approach claim a success rate approaching 90%
among those who complete their prescribed time in the therapeutic community. Opponents point to the dropout rate of more than
80% in the first 6 months and the cost of such a high-intensity
treatment to disprove its utility (9).

HARM REDUCTION

Harm reduction is a term both reviled and revered in the addiction treatment world. For a comprehensive review and explanation of the techniques of harm reduction, see Marlatt's text by that
name (10). The term describes an approach that seeks to help the
addicted individual decrease the damage being done to the self
and to those around him or her as a result of ongoing substance
use. Methadone maintenance, for example, which is discussed
later, could be viewed as a harm reduction approach. Some advo-
cates view harm reduction as a series of intermediate steps on the
road to abstinence. Others see it as a goal in itself.

A simple example of how harm reduction works, consider a patient who is drinking alcohol nightly to intoxication. His job performance is worsening with increasing episodes of absenteeism.
Although the expressed goal may be complete abstinence from alcohol, if the patient can remain abstinent during the work week so
that his job is no longer in danger, he has made a significant step
forward. If he has been drinking and driving and can be taught to
never get behind the wheel again when under the influence, he has
also decreased the risk to himself and to others. Although data are
lacking on how this applies in the dually diagnosed population, recommendations on using this approach are found in other chapters.

METHADONE MAINTENANCE

Although clearly a harm reduction technique, methadone maintenance treatment (MMT) is presented by itself as being the best
studied technique and the one for which the most data are

available. Dole and Nyswander, a physician couple, began this approach to the treatment of narcotics dependence. They believed there was something unique about opiate addicts and that they were self-medicating. They further believed that if what was missing could be replaced, the addicted individual would no longer have to use illegal narcotics. By supplying the individual with a long-acting, medicinal grade opiate, the heroin- or other opioid-dependent individual is freed of the need to buy street drugs of questionable content. Thus, this decreases criminal behavior associated with obtaining street level drugs, frequency of administration, and, therefore, the need of continually using, recovering from the most severe effects, using, recovering, and so on, so that the individual has time to pursue other activities and establish more prosocial behaviors.

In MMT, the patient is given methadone, an opiate with a long half-life. Initially, the patient must come to a clinic every day to receive the dose of medication. No take-home doses are permitted. Heroin has a short half-life so the addicted individual must use it two to four times a day to stay out of withdrawal. Methadone stops the cycle of use so that the individual can begin to move forward with life, without worry of withdrawal.

CASE 2-3

Sheila C., 39 years of age, had been shooting heroin for 15 years. She didn't even enjoy it anymore. She was a slave to the drug and she knew it. Getting high wasn't even an issue—Sheila hadn't been high in years. Although if she didn't use, she felt so bad she couldn't stand it. Repeated efforts to get clean had failed. Sheila had been on methadone now for about a year. On 90 mg, she found she didn't crave heroin. She didn't always feel as though she was going into withdrawal. For the first time in more than a decade she had a place to call home. All of her money was not going to support her habit. She even had a part-time job sacking groceries. When she had been on the street trying to get enough money for a "fix," she did not have time for a job because she had to be in constant search of money and heroin to keep out of withdrawal. It wasn't fun having to take a bus downtown every day to the clinic to drink her methadone, because she was not eligible to take any of the medication with her. But it was so much better than searching the streets for drugs and never having a roof over her head, so Sheila really didn't mind it that much.

Currently, MMT is the single most effective modality known for dealing with illicit drug use. If abstinence from all psychoactive drugs is the only acceptable endpoint in the treatment of addictive disorders (clearly, this is not reasonable in dealing with psychotic patients), then MMT is a complete failure. If, however, improving the patient's quality of life, decreasing criminal behavior, decreasing disease transmission, and encouraging other prosocial behaviors are worthwhile and acceptable goals of addiction treatment, then MMT proves to be the best proven approach to treating addictive disorders (11).

RELAPSE PREVENTION

An increasingly popular approach, relapse prevention builds on principles espoused by others, including AA. For an in-depth explanation of the principles and practice of this approach, see Marlatt's book (12). In a relapse prevention approach, individuals are taught to identify "high-risk" situations for themselves—occasions that increase their risk of using or drinking—and to develop a plan in advance for either avoiding those situations or dealing with them if they arise. They are encouraged to do these same things about people and objects. The patient is then encouraged to practice this plan. If an episode occurs during which the person uses, despite this plan, that person is encouraged to use this event as a learning experience, to look at where the plan failed or where he or she failed to observe the cues warning of the risk of relapse.

At one time, the issue of relapse was not discussed in treatment programs. It was as though treatment providers believed that talking about the subject would make it happen. The fact is, substance use disorders are defined as "chronic, relapsing conditions." Avoiding the discussion means avoiding being prepared in advance for the situation if it does happen. Patients were not prepared for how to help themselves back into recovery. Individuals who misuse substances need to be helped to understand that relapse can happen but is not inevitable. In addition, relapse should not be used as an excuse for continuing to use.

CASE 2-4

Ms. H., age 43 years, had been abstinent of alcohol and other substances for 8 months until her birthday. As she had for many years, she bought a six pack of beer and, on returning home, immediately drank two. Realizing that this was putting herself at risk of resuming her previous, heavy alcohol use, she poured the remainder down the sink.

Ms. H.'s counselor could approach this situation in one of two ways. In one scenario, the counselor could express disappointment in her and castigate her for her weakness; in the other, congratulate her for exerting some control over the situation and rejecting further use. Then, the counselor could encourage her to think about other upcoming high-risk events and begin developing a plan for how to avoid using in the future.

Contrary to popular belief, experience shows that even individuals who are physiologically dependent on psychoactive substances can stop themselves from using and can exert some control over continuing to use if they stop soon enough. A problem with the concept that the addicted individual is "powerless" once succumbing to the temptation to even sample the drug of choice is that this becomes a self-fulfilling prophecy. Patients who are convinced they cannot stop, do not try to stop.

Throughout the remainder of this text, focus is on a variety of therapeutic techniques (and combinations of several) the treatment provider will be encouraged to use when working with psychiatrically ill patients with comorbid substance use disorders. Rather than working in one theoretic framework, most clinicians who work extensively with the dually diagnosed find themselves to be confirmed pragmatists: find out what works for the particular patient, and use it. No one thing works for everyone.

REFERENCES

1. Ridgely MS, Goldman HH, Willenbring M. Barriers to the care of persons with dual diagnoses: organizational and financing issues. *Schizophr Bull* 1990;16:123–132.
2. Weiss RD, Najavits LM. Overview of treatment modalities for dual diagnosis patients. In: Kranzler HR, Rounsaville BJ, eds. *Dual diagnosis and treatment: substance abuse and comorbid medical and psychiatric disorders.* New York: Marcel Dekker, 1998:87–105.
3. McLellan AT, Luborsky L, Woody GE, et al. Predicting response to drug and alcohol treatments: role of psychiatric severity. *Arch Gen Psychiatry* 1983;40:620–625.
4. Drake RE, McHugo GJ, Noordsy DL. Treatment of alcoholism among schizophrenic outpatients: four-year outcomes. *Am J Psychiatry* 1993;150:328–329.
5. Kofoed L, Kania J, Walsh T, et al. Outpatient treatment of patients with substance abuse and coexisting psychiatric disorders. *Am J Psychiatry* 1986;143:867–872.
6. Hellerstein DJ, Meehan B. Outpatient group therapy for schizophrenic substance abusers. *Am J Psychiatry* 1987;144:1337–1339.
7. Ries RK, Ellingson T. A pilot assessment at one month of seventeen dual diagnosis patients. *Hospital and Community Psychiatry* 1989;41:1230–1233.
8. Galanter M. *Network therapy for alcohol and drug abuse.* New York: Guilford Press, 1993.
9. Schuckit MA. Rehabilitation. In: Shuckit MA. *Drug and alcohol abuse: a clinical guide to diagnosis and treatment.* New York: Kluwer Academic/Plenum Publishers, 2000:332.
10. Marlatt GA, ed. *Harm reduction: pragmatic strategies for managing high risk behaviors.* New York: Guilford Press, 1998.
11. Bell J, Zador D. A risk-benefit analysis of methadone maintenance treatment. *Drug Saf* 2000;22(3):179–190.
12. Marlatt GA, Gordon JR, eds. *Relapse prevention: maintenance strategies in the treatment of addictive behaviors.* New York, Guilford Press, 1985.

Evaluation and Goal Setting

1. Approach to the addicted individual must be nonjudgmental
2. Basic questions in evaluation of the addicted patient
   a. How and when got started
   b. What have you tried? What have you been dependent on?
   c. Current amount using
   d. Context of use: With whom? What? When? Where? Why?
   e. Upside and downside to using
   f. Route of administration
   g. Number of times attempting to quit and relative success
   h. Why quit now?
   i. Longest period of continuous abstinence and how this was achieved
   j. Number of times in treatment, whether or not this was beneficial and why?
   k. Consequences of using
3. Medical evaluation
4. Steps in the treatment of the dually diagnosed patient
   a. Detoxification as indicated
   b. Psychiatric stabilization
   c. Engagement
   d. Goal setting and establishment of abstinence
   e. Clarification of myths regarding substances of abuse and of psychiatric illnesses
   f. Establishment and rehearsal of a personal relapse prevention plan

---

It would seem obvious to the point of unnecessary to say that the addicted patient must be approached in a nonjudgmental fashion. Yet, substance use disorders tend to bring out the worst in healthcare providers. Much of this may result from the fact that, in training, students seldom see the successes. Instead, they see only the repeat failures who appear sicker each time they return for care.

In looking at other medical conditions, however, periods of relapse and improvement are the norm. For example, it is not uncommon for persons with hypertension occasionally to eat salted popcorn and diabetics to eat cheesecake, although each knows that such behavior worsens the specific condition. Yet, such behaviors seldom arouse the anger in us that the alcohol-dependent individual who falls off the wagon for a weekend can arouse.

The diabetic's obesity is recognized as a primary factor in hyperglycemia, likewise the salty diet the hypertensive insists on consuming. At some point, however, we recognize that the disease often takes on a life of its own, irrespective of dietary control and weight loss, and tend not to pass judgment. Although willing to forgive such behaviors, we ignore the fact that the exact same principles apply to those with addictive disorders.

Just as with the diabetic who stops sneaking cookies because he does not like the sick feeling he or she gets, and the hypertensive who avoids potato chips because it causes headaches, alcoholics can also come to learn to change their behaviors, to their betterment. No one wants to be diabetic, hypertensive, or alcoholic. Changing behaviors, however, takes time.

EVALUATING THE DUALLY DIAGNOSED PATIENT

Any thorough psychiatric evaluation should include questions regarding both mental illness and substance use. Mental health professionals, however, often overlook the latter. Questions specific to each psychiatric disorder will not be covered here. For this, the reader is referred to the *Diagnostic and Statistical Manual of Mental Disorders* (1) for the specific criteria of the various disorders covered. Following is the minimal information necessary to assess the substance misusing patient and begin to develop a plan for treatment (Table 3-1).

How and When Got Started

Adolescent experimentation with substances is arguably a normal behavior. The *chronic* use of alcohol and other substances by teens, however, is often symptomatic of other psychopathology (2,3). It is clear that most young people who try mood-altering drugs do not go on to develop substance use disorders. It is also clear that the younger age one starts to use psychoactive substances and the more often one uses them, the more likely one is to develop a frank dependence on a psychoactive substance. The answer to the question of when the individual began to use substances can help to establish whether a substance use disorder is primary or secondary, which helps to guide treatment. Memory is often flawed, however, and it is often difficult or even impossible to assess accurately which came first—the substance use disorder or another mood or psychiatric condition.

It is also helpful to know if the individual started using a year ago and only now feels "hooked" or started using 30 years ago and has never been abstinent. Not only does the answer to this question have prognostic value, but it will guide treatment recommendations as well. The recent user could well be advised to participate in an outpatient program, whereas the latter user would likely best be served in a long-term inpatient facility.

How the individual got started is also helpful to know, which will provide a clue to the individual's strengths and weaknesses. Men tend to start because their peers are using substances, whereas women tend to begin because of a relationship with a significant other who is doing so (4,5). A female patient whose boyfriend started her using will need help with her substance use, as well as with her object choices and issues of autonomy.

How Often and How Much?

It is not necessary to use a substance every day to have a substantial problem with the substance. Some alcohol-dependent individuals begin drinking in the morning (an "eye opener") and keep a drink going throughout the day. Others limit their use to a specific time of day, perhaps after work, or to weekends only, yet can consume a large amount of alcohol during that time, resulting in social, occupational, or physical sequelae and withdrawal symptoms. Crack cocaine users often use their drug in a "binge" fashion. They consume a large quantity of their drug in one episode, ending when the money or the drug runs out, followed by 3 or 4 days of

Table 3-1. Assessing the substance misuser

1. How and when started
    Age of onset
    Length of time using
    (Normative behavior *vs.* symptom of more pathologic condition)
2. What have you tried? What have you used?
    (Differentiating between physiologic dependence
    and experimentation)
3. Do you think you were ever "hooked" on anything?
    If yes, have you overcome this dependence on other substances?
    (Past history of success can be used as reassurance for a patient
    who is becoming discouraged. Can also be used by the patient
    to deny need for help.)
4. How much and how often are you currently using?
    (Not necessary to use daily to still have a pathologic pattern of use)
    (How much should prompt question regarding how the habit is
    supported or involvement in criminal activity.)
    (Stress of legal involvement may keep patient from concentrating
    on recovery issues.)
5. Context of use: With whom? What? When? Where? Why?
    (With whom: helps establish the patient's peer group or
    knowledge of social network and how difficult it will be
    for patient to avoid being around using people.)
    (When and where: times of day may be particularly difficult for
    some people and the "where" is the "places" part of "people,
    places, and things" to avoid.)
    ("Why": start focusing the patient on what he or she wishes to
    experience or achieve when using or beginning to look at
    alternate means to achieve the same things.)
6. Benefits of using: as above—what do you achieve or experience,
    if anything, as a result of using?
7. Downside to "using": the counterpoint to above—what are the
    negative consequences, if any, that using has caused?
8. How have you used (i.e., IV, snort, oral, intranasal)?
    (Important in directing interviewer to issues regarding possible
    disease transmission and other health risks.)
9. Have you ever tried to quit? How many times? What happened?
    (Helps the interviewer to capitalize on past successes and
    develop plans to avoid previous pitfalls.)
10. Why quit now?
    (Helps to understand the motivation for change and assess how
    realistic the individual's expectations are for change.)
11. Longest period of continuous abstinence? How did you achieve
    this? Why or how did you get started again?
12. Have you ever been in treatment? How many times? Was it
    helpful? Why or why not?
13. Any consequences of using?

abstinence before the drug use starts again. Heroin-dependent individuals, on the other hand, typically use two to four times per day to avoid withdrawal symptoms.

The answer to this question will help the treatment provider to determine the level of care the individual needs and whether or not detoxification services will be needed. The individual who daily drinks a couple of glasses of wine at lunch and three or four beers in the evening, does not miss work, has no health consequences as a result of it, and is not a worry to his or her spouse is still drinking more than is recommended. This person might benefit from a brief intervention from the family physician and information on recommended levels of alcohol consumption, health risks, and alternative drinking behaviors. The person who drinks all day every day, has had seizures when attempting to stop, and has had an esophageal hemorrhage during a drinking episode needs hospitalization and a controlled detoxification followed by inpatient rehabilitation, if possible.

What Have You Tried? Used?

Differentiating between *trying* and *using* is not "hairsplitting," and individuals with drug use disorders tend to understand the difference. Again, adolescent experimentation with some drugs (e.g., trying something once or twice, typically the ones friends are using) is not abnormal. "Trying" *vs.* "using" can have prognostic significance. Individuals who have used large amounts of crystal methamphetamine or 3,4-methylenedioxymethamphetamine (MDMA; ecstasy) may display long-term or even permanent neurochemical changes, whereas those who have simply tried it a few times may not, although insufficient data exist to say this with certainty (6).

How Many Times Did You Use the Substance?

Did you ever think you were hooked? If so (given that the individual is no longer using this substance), how did you stop?

This can have some importance to the individual. On the one hand, the individual who has "stopped on (his or her) own" may use this as an excuse to avoid seeking or accepting help. ("I don't need any help stopping alcohol. I can stop anytime I want"), or ("I don't need any help stopping. I've stopped other things. I'm just not going to use it any more."). On the other hand, it can be encouraging to the individual to be reminded that he or she has done it before and can be helped to "do it again," to help overcome the feeling of hopelessness experienced in ongoing addiction.

CONTEXT OF USE—CURRENT

In 12-step programs, individuals attempting to recover from a substance use disorder are admonished to be aware of "people, places, and things." This admonition means avoid (a) being in situations and around people with whom they have used their drugs of choice or with whom they associate the using life; (b) places where they have used or bought their drugs; and (c) objects (e.g., a pipe or a beer bottle) that are reminders of their past substance use. Any or all of these factors can act as a trigger to start using again. In addition, each is unique for the individual, although common themes can exist.

Examples

People, obviously, are going to be personal. However, living with someone who uses makes recovery difficult for the individual, especially if that someone uses at home. Constant confrontation with another's substance of choice can be a setup for failure. Just being around someone who is "getting high" can mitigate against success, especially if the recovering person begins to feel left out, unhappy, hopeless, or that he or she "deserves" to get high.

Places

Some places are obvious, such as bars where using an intoxicant is both accepted and encouraged. Early in recovery, some individuals will stay in such places to "test" themselves or because this is where their friends spend their time. Although nothing is absolute, such a limited social milieu and the constant presence of substance use can present a significant obstacle to abstinence.

Things

Things can be relapse cues; that is, circumstances that act as a trigger for the individual to resume using psychoactive substances are personal. Individuals attempting recovery should be encouraged to identify their own personal cues in order to avoid putting themselves in high-risk situations. Despite the personal nature of relapse cues, some common themes can be found. For some cocaine users, for example, money, white powder, or the sight of paraphernalia can act as triggers. A certain time of day (the time they would normally being drinking, for example, can be a trigger for some alcohol abusers).

Why?

Why is not merely a philosophical question, but rather, an opportunity to begin pointing the individual in the direction of personal expectations as a result of using. In general, people have a reason for what they do, and the reasons can differ widely. Some people use to be part of the crowd. Others start out of curiosity. Some want to escape from their current life or simply feel "different." The initial reason for using and for continued use, however, often differs. The "why" here is the first examination of the patient's motivation for using, that is, to begin to determine what expectation exists for using. It is common for patients to indicate they continue to use out of fear of withdrawal or because they are unable to feel "normal" without their drug of choice. Another way of asking this question is: What is it you are looking for or what do you want to have happen as a result of using? Some people cannot answer this question—using their drug of choice is so much a part of them that they have never considered being otherwise. Others have very specific expectations or experiences they want to achieve as a result of using: relief of tension, to change their mood, to help them sleep, and so on. For others (e.g., long-time heroin users), the answer may be that they no longer enjoy the drug and they are unable to achieve a "high," but they feel so bad if they do not use they have to keep using. These users are enslaved to their one-time friend. The person who cannot articulate an expectation for use requires more help in identifying relapse triggers. The individual who can verbalize expectations, can then be asked to consider alternative ways of achieving the same goal.

See Chapter 16 for examples of "Motivation for Use" charts. In this exercise, the individual is instructed to look at what it is he or she *wants* the drug of choice to do for him or her, what this drug of choice actually *does,* and whether the two are the same. If they are the same, in what other ways can the same effect be obtained? If they are not the same, can the individual begin to develop strategies to effectively achieve those goals?

How Have You Used?

As noted in Chapter 4, substances can be used in a variety of ways. Riskiest, of course, is intravenous (i.v.) use. All substance users, but especially those who admit to a history of i.v. drug use should be asked questions regarding risk of acquired immunodeficiency syndrome (AIDS) and hepatitis and a referral to a general medical clinic for evaluation. Questions should include information on needle sharing. Intravenous drug use also implies a degree of risk-taking that snorting, drinking, or smoking a drug does not. Each route of use is associated with its own risks and should prompt questions specific to that particular pattern of use. Drinking should cause the questioner to ask about vomiting blood and passing blood in the stool, for example. Snorting should prompt questions about nosebleeds and sinus infections (some of which can be serious).

Have You Ever Tried to Quit?

The answer to "Have you ever tried to quit?" can be double edged. On the one hand, the shorter the period of time one has been using, the easier it is to stop. On the other hand, individuals typically attempt to stop any substance use several times before they actually succeed. Further, the individuals who have experienced multiple treatment failures may become discouraged and begin to believe that it is impossible to improve their condition. Nevertheless, it is helpful to know if the individual has tried to stop before and what happened. How successful was that person? If he or she succeeded for awhile, how did he or she remain successful for that period of time? What happened to cause resumed use? Answers to these questions help the therapist to know something about pitfalls to help the patient develop a strategy for avoiding them in the future.

Longest Period of Continuous Abstinence?

Again, it is helpful to know something about the individual's relative degree of success (or lack thereof) in maintaining any degree of abstinence, to gain a better understanding of how easy or difficult it had been for that person. It is also helpful, once again, to know how the patient has accomplished this. There is considerable difference between someone who stayed sober for 2 years while incarcerated and the one who did the same thing while living in the community and supporting self and family. For each, however, it is helpful to know the circumstances of the relapse, which may help the individual to focus on high-risk situations and a way to avoid them.

The "Downside" and "Upside" to Using

Individuals coming into treatment often avoid talking about the benefits of their use. When asked: "What does (your substance) do for you?" they say, "nothing," expecting a trap. They feel they may be criticized for naming anything positive to their use. But people use for a reason. Sometimes the reason is as simple as they enjoy it. With an understanding of the motivation behind the use, the treatment provider can work with the patient to develop an individualized approach to achieving abstinence. Then alternate behaviors for achieving the desired result can be found.

Likewise, the individual in treatment is there for a reason. What is it? What is the motivation for seeking treatment? What is the "downside" to using that is causing the individual to come for treatment? It could be legal, family, or peer pressure, or the realization current substance use is ruining his or her life and health. Regardless of the reason, it is helpful for the treatment provider to understand why the patient is there in order to help formulate a plan of how to approach the individual's problem in the most effective manner.

"Just saying no" as the alternate strategy to using is not sufficient. Patients must develop new behaviors to replace their old using habits. One strategy may be attendance at 12-step meetings, which can replace time previously spent using and with people who used with time and people likewise attempting to gain abstinence. For others, it may be developing a hobby, volunteering, or exercise. Any positive strategy that helps individuals avoid people, places, and things that they associate with using should be encouraged. The only unacceptable choice is to do nothing. If nothing is done to fill the void (i.e., no new behaviors are developed), the individual is likely to fail.

MEDICAL EVALUATION

Volumes exist regarding the medical needs of addicted persons and such information is beyond the scope of this book. Nevertheless, the clinician is advised to keep a few important issues in mind. Clearly, a complete history and physical examination with a battery of screening tests to rule out a number of substance-related medical conditions would be the ideal course to follow in working with a substance-misusing patient. Reality, however, tends to differ. Many outpatient clinics dealing with either addicted populations or psychiatric populations lack space or funds for other than the most rudimentary evaluation: blood pressure, pulse, and referral out for laboratory testing if the physician who rotates through the clinic deems this desirable.

At the very least, keep in mind that individuals with addiction problems tend to be nutritionally deprived and at increased risk of infectious diseases. Drinkers tend not to eat when they are drinking and when they do eat, do not absorb all the nutrients they need. If a full medical workup is not possible, suggest that the patient take a multiple vitamin with additional thiamine and folic acid. Much information exists to show that smoking crack cocaine is associated with increased high-risk sexual activity, human immunodeficiency virus (HIV) infection, and other sexually transmitted diseases. Testing for these diseases would be of benefit. The risks associated with i.v. drug use are extensive and well known. Screening for infectious diseases known to occur with this form of drug use is also advisable.

STEPS IN THE TREATMENT OF THE DUALLY DIAGNOSED PATIENT

The steps in the treatment of the dually diagnosed patient are fluid. The treatment process, especially with chronically mentally ill patients, will be punctuated by advances and backsliding, disappearance from treatment, and reappearance with requests for help. Generally, the necessary steps are (a) detoxification, as indicated; (b) psychiatric stabilization; (c) ongoing efforts at engagement; (d) establishment of abstinence; (e) goal setting; (f) clarifying and correcting myths and beliefs about drugs of abuse; (g) clarifying and correcting myths about psychiatric illnesses and medications; and (h) establishment and rehearsal of a personal relapse prevention plan (Fig. 3-1).

Detoxification

Chapter 5 addresses the issue of detoxification.

Goal Setting

Whose goals? Once evaluation is complete, the next step is to establish the goals of treatment. One of the challenges of treating the dually diagnosed individual is to establish goals that are personally meaningful to the patient. Traditionally, addiction treatment programs have dictated the goal as abstinence now, abstinence later, and this above all else. For the mental health treatment provider, medication compliance and stabilization of the psychiatric disorder are common goals. The problem, however, is that the patient may have neither in mind. In fact, the patient may have no interest in treatment at all if he or she is

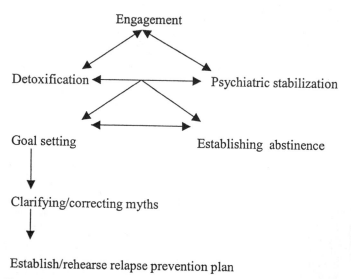

Figure 3-1.

coming to treatment under duress, by pressure either from the legal system or family. Thus, the challenge for the therapist is to help the patient find a reason to be there and establish goals that are personally worth working toward. That is, the therapist must help the patient develop a motivation for ongoing treatment. For a comprehensive review of improving client motivation, see *Motivational Interviewing* by Miller and Rollnick on how to apply it to addicted populations (7).

Arguably, the goal of treatment should be multifaceted and include improving the individual's overall quality of life. In addition to reducing and perhaps eventually eliminating substance use, treatment should include promoting prosocial behaviors such as employment, a stable living arrangement, nonabusive relationships, and the absence of legal problems. Complete and total abstinence from all psychoactive substances may be neither attainable nor desirable, especially for those individuals who will require medication to stabilize their psychiatric conditions. Especially in dealing with the dually diagnosed, it is reasonable to view "recovery" on a continuum.

CASE 3-1

Mike L., 34 years of age, has schizophrenia. His life for 8 years was a series of hospitalizations for exacerbations of psychosis, incarcerations for being drunk and disorderly or for threatening behavior, and periods of homelessness. He would spend all of his disability checks on alcohol and cocaine. Since becoming engaged in treatment, he has had only three hospitalizations in 12 months. From 24 of 24 drug screens positive for cocaine the previous year, only 2 of 14 were positive while in treatment. Where he had never been able to maintain an apartment because he always spent his money on drugs before his rent was paid, he has held onto the same place for 7 months.

Mike is an individual for whom the harm reduction approach has much meaning. Perhaps he has not achieved the goals most desirable to the caregiver, but he has not failed to make progress, either. He can be applauded for his successes and the circumstances around his hospitalizations used as information from which to learn. What should he do differently in the future to avoid needing to go into the hospital again?

Any care provider can do a better job with an understanding of why a stated goal is important to the patient. A stated goal should be explored, rather than taken at face value. For example, treatment-wise clients often offer that "abstinence" is their goal. Although this might be desirable for the patient, it is reasonable to ask "why?" Is this said to please the clinician, or is the patient sincere about the goal? If sincere, what has happened as a result of using that makes it desirable to stop? What is the patient hoping will happen if he or she stops using? Is the patient setting self up for disappointment and possible relapse by establishing an unattainable goal? For example, does the patient believe that marital problems will end when drinking ends? If the spouse still leaves even though the patient is sober, this may hasten a relapse. On the other hand, if the patient wants to quit drinking because of being ashamed of being hung over every day and wants to eliminate that feeling, that patient can feel proud of waking up clear headed.

Common goals presented by dually diagnosed clients include (a) gaining the ability to control their drinking or drug use; (b) to satisfy the legal system or family; (c) no idea whatsoever why they are there or what might be accomplished by their participation in the dually diagnosed program; and (d) goals that appear to be tangential or unrelated to their dually diagnosed participation (an example of which is given below).

Controlled Use

While "controlling" the use of a substance runs counter to traditional addiction treatment goals, it is worth exploring what this means to the individual. The client who presents this as a goal is indicating an awareness that the substance use is causing some problems. This is a perfect opening for the therapist to determine from the client what these problems might have been, what controlled use means, and why this is important. It is important for the treatment provider to know, and to let the patient know, that controlled use is not the most common outcome, although some limited literature suggests it is possible (8,9). Nevertheless, it is reasonable to explore the client's stated goal and why that goal is important to the patient. It is not at all uncommon for clients (usually through personal experience) to find that they rapidly increase their substance use once they start, and to embrace abstinence as a necessary goal.

To Satisfy the Legal (or Other) System

This goal can be reframed. For example:

"What will happen (e.g., legally, family-wise, etc.) if you participate?"
"I'll be kicked out, go to jail, and so on, if I don't come here."
Becomes: "I will remain at home, in good graces with the family, out of jail, and so forth."

No Idea

This is often the response given by someone who is resistant or who, perhaps justifiably, feels coerced into treatment. It can also be the response of a very concrete thinking individual with a thought disorder. This patient should be encouraged to continue in treatment to explore whether or not something may be of benefit as a result of attending.

Goals That Appear Unrelated or Tangential to Treatment

Clinicians working with severely mentally ill clients become accustomed to having goals offered that do not appear to be a primary function of treatment. With some imagination, however, it is possible to bring the goal into relevance, as in the case below.

CASE 3-2

Mr. D., on being asked what he wanted to accomplish by participating in the dually diagnosed group, stated "A puppy." Mr. D. had schizophrenia and, except when using cocaine, tends to be withdrawn and asocial. His thinking is remarkable for being

very concrete and often delusional. It is the therapist's job to
clarify why this goal is meaningful to the client: What have been
the impediments to accomplishing this goal in the past? How has
his substance use affected its attainment? What is his under-
standing of what the stated goal may mean?

Therapist:

Why would you like to have a puppy?
Have you ever had a puppy before? Why or why not?
What happened to it?
How much money do you spend on cocaine?
How much money do you get each month?
What does a puppy need?
They need shots, someone at home every day, food, a license, train-
  ing, companionship.
How often are you hospitalized, incarcerated, or homeless each
  month?
When you are hospitalized, incarcerated, or homeless who will
  take care of the puppy?
If you spend $__ amount of money per month on cocaine, how
  much does that leave for feeding and caring for the puppy?

Mr. D.'s stated goal was recorded for him, and revisited frequently while in treatment. As he slowly decreased and finally
discontinued his cocaine use, he was able to see that he would
have enough money to care for a puppy and did, in fact, purchase
one. Thus, a seemingly tangential goal can be reframed in such
a way that it is attainable within the treatment program.

PSYCHIATRIC STABILIZATION

Especially with the patient who is actively using substances of
abuse, psychiatric stabilization is an ongoing and sometimes frustrating task. A mistake commonly made in the past was to withhold patients' medications when they were drinking or using other
drugs. Clearly, this only serves to further destabilize the patient's
already tenuous condition.

Choosing the correct (safe) medication is critical. (The chapters
to follow deal with the issues of medications and their potential
interactions with substances of abuse.) When the patient is in a
controlled environment (e.g., a hospital or halfway house), the
concern lessens about the patient using a drug of choice in addition to prescribed psychotropic medication. It can still occur, but
the chances are lower than if the patient is out on the street.

Increasingly, however, insurance will not cover inpatient stays
for detoxification and treatment of substance misuse in the absence of a medical crisis, and facilities for placing patients are decreasing in number. Thus, clinicians are faced with the task of
treating patients who truly need their help, but could potentially
develop toxic reactions by combining prescription medications
with drugs of abuse.

Engagement

Engagement is the process of developing a trusting, accepting
relationship with the patient and creating a "buy-in" by the

patient of the treatment process. Engaging chronically mentally ill clients in the treatment process can be very protracted because of the patient's lack of comprehension, poor compliance, rejection of diagnosis, and many other factors. Therapists working in the mental health system realize that consistency and time are essential to patient engagement—a process that cannot be rushed.

During the period of engagement and whenever possible, it is helpful to remove the patient from the environment in which substances of abuse are used. This does not necessarily mean institutionalization. It may mean relocation with nonusing friends or family. If this is not possible, it may be helpful to pair the patient with nonusing others to assist the individual in an environment where others are using psychoactive substances. This could consist of friends, family, members of 12-step groups, churches or synagogues, and anyone else devoted to helping the patient obtain and maintain abstinence. Sometimes, neither of these efforts is possible and the only option may be to keep the patient coming back to the treatment facility and out of the home environment as much as possible.

Clarifying and Correcting Myths About Drugs of Abuse and Psychiatric Illnesses and Medications

It is important to find out what the patient understands about his or her mental illness and drug of abuse. Those who work with addicted individuals know that, although users of street drugs often have an amazing knowledge of ways to "get high," they also often subscribe to some grossly inaccurate beliefs about their drugs of choice and how they work. In addition, individuals with mental illnesses often have an inaccurate understanding of what they can expect from their illnesses and how they will run their course. Some patients believe it is a personal failing if they are depressed, anxious, or hear voices. It is important to correct any misunderstandings and make sure the individual is working with accurate information (Table 3-2).

It is also important for the therapist to work with factual information, not with scare tactics. A therapist loses credibility if he or she suggests that the use of any marijuana or alcohol—no matter how little—inevitably results in a recurrence of symptoms and rehospitalization and the patient knows from personal experience that this is not the case.

Some commonly held myths:

I can't be an alcoholic, I only drink beer.
Alcohol isn't a drug.
Ecstasy won't hurt you.
If you can hold your liquor, you can't be an alcoholic.
Alcohol helps you sleep.
Marijuana has no health risks.
Once you're an alcoholic or drug addict, you can never use even a
  little bit (of your drug of choice) or you'll lose all control.
You can be cured of schizophrenia or bipolar illness.
You should stop taking your medication if you drink or do drugs.
If you have a mental illness or if you're an alcoholic, your kids will
  have a mental illness or will be an alcoholic too.

Table 3-2. Myths and realities

Myth	Reality
I can't be an alcoholic; I only drink beer	Although the Surgeon General's warning regarding pregnancy and alcohol will be on the label, beer bottles, especially if they come from a case, may not indicate they have an alcohol content, helping to promote a beer drinker's denial that beer is an alcoholic beverage. In truth, beer-a-holics often truly do not realize that they can develop cirrhosis and die of alcohol-related illnesses and never have touched a drop of hard liquor or wine in their lives.
Alcohol isn't a drug	Because nicotine and alcohol use is legal, heavy misusers of both often feel a need to set themselves apart from users of other substances. They look down on "drug addicts," but can forgive their own problem.
Ecstasy won't hurt you	Unfortunately, few hard data have been available until recently to refute this piece of misinformation. Increasingly, it appears that heavy exposure to ecstasy may have long-term and, possibly, permanent sequelae.
If you can hold your liquor, you won't be an alcoholic	Being able to "drink everyone under the table" was once an admired trait. Now, however, genetic studies have shown that individuals least responsive to the effects of alcohol are actually at an increased risk of developing long-term problems as a result of use.
Alcohol helps you sleep	A long-held, but inaccurate notion, alcohol suppresses rapid eye movement sleep, resulting in fitful, unrestful sleep.
Marijuana has no health risks	Data are still equivocal, but it appears that respiratory problems may be worsened. In addition, concern exists that some types of cancers increase in long-term, heavy marijuana users.
Once you're addicted, you can never use even a little bit or you will lose control	Studies show that some addicted individuals can and do return to controlled use after a period of abstinence. Others find that they can use a small amount of their substance of choice without trouble. Once past a critical point, however, which is idiosyncratic, they do appear to lose control. Don't let the individual use a slip as an excuse to keep using!

Continued

Table 3-2. *Continued*

Myth	Reality
You can be cured of schizophrenia or bipolar illness	Both of these illnesses are heavily genetically influenced. To is date, no "cure" exists for either, although both are treatable with a number of available medications.
You should stop your medication if you drink or use drugs	Because substance use is virtually guaranteed to worsen the course of psychiatric illnesses, this is a time when medication should adamantly be continued.
If you have a substance dependence or mental illness, then your kids will too	The risk is increased for both, because both conditions are genetically influenced. By no means is there a 100% relationship, and no guarantee exists for either condition.

The therapist needs to be able to address these and other erroneous beliefs the patient may have or be willing to admit a lack of knowledge and find the correct answers. Informational sheets for patients are found in Chapter 16.

ESTABLISHMENT AND REHEARSAL OF A PERSONAL RELAPSE PREVENTION PLAN

As discussed, cues to relapse, the "people, places, and things" that 12-step programs talk about are different for different people. It is beneficial for each patient to identify personal relapse cues, to develop a plan for how to avoid relapse when feeling it is about to occur, and what to do if it does. If the patient waits until the occasion presents to figure out what to do, it is too late. Some simple and widely used techniques are to always carry an index card with the names and phone numbers of one's AA or NA sponsor and a few other group members who can be called if the patient feels the urge to use. Another is to have a list of consequences that have occurred as a result of past experiences with using (e.g., medical, legal, marital, and so on) to help act as a deterrent to using. Some people find that having a list of places to go as well as how to get there quickly, or money in a sealed envelope so they can get away from a high-risk situation is helpful. Basically, whatever the individual feels to be most beneficial should be established well in advance of the time such is needed, and practiced so that the routine is familiar.

REFERENCES

1. American Psychiatric Association. *Diagnostic and statistical manual of mental disorders,* IV. Washington, DC: American Psychiatric Association, 1994.

2. White HR, Xie M, Thompson W, et al. Psychopathology as a predictor of adolescent drug use trajectories. *Psychol Addict Behav* 2001;15(3):210–218.
3. Sussman S, Dent CW, Galaif ER. The correlates of substance abuse and dependence among adolescents at high risk for drug abuse. *J Subst Abuse* 1997;9:241–255.
4. Wilsnack SC. Patterns and trends in women's drinking: recent findings and some implications for prevention. In: Howard JM, Martin SE, Mail PD, et al., eds. *Women and alcohol: issues for prevention and research,* Vol. Research monograph No. 32. Bethesda, MD: National Institutes of Health, 1996.
5. Demers A, Bisson J, Palluy J. Wives' convergence with their husbands' alcohol use: social conditions as mediators. *J Stud Alcohol* 1999;60:368–377.
6. Buchert R, Obrocki J, Thomasius R, et al. Long-term effects of 'ecstasy' abuse on the human brain studied by FDG PET. *Nucl Med Commun* 2001;22(8):889–897.
7. Miller WR, Rollnick S. *Motivational interviewing: preparing people to change addictive behavior.* New York: Guilford Press, 1991.
8. Sobell MB, Sobell LC. Controlled drinking after 25 years: how important was the great debate? *Addiction* 1995;90(9):1149–1153.
9. Mills KC, Sobell MB, Schaefer HH. Training social drinking as an alternative to abstinence for alcoholics. *Behav Res Ther* 1971;2(1):18–27.

4

Reviewing the Action of Substances of Abuse

1. Nicotine
   a. Most widely used of all substances of abuse
   b. Dirty drug with multiple substances associated with it
   c. Both negative and positive effects on the body
   d. Pregnancy: use during pregnancy increases risk of spontaneous abortion, smaller neonates, and sudden infant death syndrome
   e. Psychiatric implications: increased use among individuals with psychiatric conditions. Cessation of use can worsen some of these conditions
2. Alcohol
   a. Men and women metabolize and distribute alcohol differently in the body
   b. As with nicotine, can have both negative and positive effects on the body
   c. Behavioral effects are unpredictable
   d. Pregnancy: multiple deleterious effects on a continuum
   e. Medical: can cause damage to every organ system
   f. Withdrawal can occur on a continuum
      i. Benign to life-threatening
      ii. Most severe form is delirium tremens with risk of fatality
3. Cannabis
   a. "Dirty" drug with multiple chemicals contained in it
   b. Effect dependent on user's expectations
   c. No lethal dose known
   d. Psychiatric result is variable, from mild euphoria to paranoia and psychosis
   e. Pregnancy: data limited and affected by typical presence of nicotine
   f. Withdrawal: medically insignificant but can be protracted and uncomfortable
4. Stimulants
   a. Cocaine used as prototype
   b. Causes general autonomic arousal
   c. Multiple cardiovascular consequences can occur
   d. Pregnancy: primarily cardiovascular consequences; developmental consequences to neonate unclear
   e. Psychiatric consequences: suicidal depression, paranoia, psychosis
   f. Withdrawal: medically insignificant; risk of suicide early after period of cocaine use
5. Opioids
   a. Euphoriants
   b. Medical consequences generally result of mode of administration
   c. Psychiatric consequences negligible
   d. Pregnancy: mild effects; withdrawal in the neonate
   e. Withdrawal
      i. Dehydration common
      ii. Medication regimen popular
      iii. Seldom life-threatening in healthy individual

For an outstanding review of many of the common and unusual substances of abuse, see the books by Richard Rudgley, one of which is referenced at the end of this chapter.

NICOTINE: BRIEF HISTORY

In general, nicotine is considered a stimulant, although at high doses hallucinations are possible. The South American Indians recognized the latter property and used nicotine for this purpose. Tobacco, the source of nicotine, is native to the Western Hemisphere. Records of its use date back more than 11,000 years. Now known worldwide, nicotine was brought to Europe in the 16th century (1).

Nicotine is among the most widely used drugs of abuse. Currently, 60 million people in the United States are cigarette smokers. This is 28% of all Americans more than 12 years of age, and 28% of the female population and 31% of the male population. The percentage of men using cigarettes has declined steadily from a high of 43% in 1985, whereas it has increased among women over the same time period. Tobacco use causes more than 1,100 deaths per day in the U.S., and it is the single most preventable cause of premature death in the Western Hemisphere. Of every five deaths in the United States, one is attributable to the use of tobacco. It is estimated that nearly half of all regular tobacco users die as a result of their smoking (2–6).

Absorption and Elimination

Nicotine, in the form of tobacco, can be smoked, chewed, or taken intranasally as "snuff." Tobacco is a "very dirty" drug. That is, when it is smoked, a large number of substances, possibly in excess of 4,000 different compounds, are introduced into the host besides just nicotine. These chemicals include acetone, arsenic, hydrogen cyanide, and carbon monoxide, among others (7). Nicotine is rapidly absorbed into the lungs by smoking and crosses into the bloodstream as well when chewed or "snuffed." Most smokers tend to adjust their smoking to maintain what is, for them, a normal level of nicotine. Individual variation in metabolism can influence how much an individual smokes. Data show that when the urine is acidified, thereby increasing the rate of nicotine excretion, smokers use more tobacco to maintain their nicotine levels (8).

Physiologic Response

The immediate effect of the drug is to stimulate discharge of norepinephrine from the adrenal cortex, causing a generalized stimulation of the central nervous system (CNS). In response to this, glucose is released which, as it drops, causes depression, fatigue, and the overwhelming desire to use again. The noradrenergic release results in increased heart rate, vasoconstriction, and concomitant increase in blood pressure. Among other effects, this rise in blood pressure can result in increased cardiac pressure, enlargement of the heart, and delay in wound healing. Despite its numerous drawbacks, good evidence indicates that nicotine use improves performance on some cognitive tests. For some time, it was assumed that when smokers claimed to "think better" when they smoked, they were simply rationalizing. It is now clear that nicotine does exert positive cognitive effects, even on nonsmokers and never smokers (9–14).

Pregnancy and Lactation

Of pregnant women, 20% smoke during pregnancy and nearly a third of this number continue to do so throughout gestation.

Studies have shown that tobacco use in pregnancy results in an increased risk of spontaneous abortion as well as decrease in weight and length of the newborn, but no morphologic abnormalities and no change in gestational age (5,15–18). Nicotine and its metabolite cotinine are present in breast milk. The impact of this finding on the neonate, however, is not clear (19,20). It is well established that maternal smoking during pregnancy is a risk factor for sudden infant death syndrome (SIDS), with the risk increasing in a dose-dependent fashion (21,22).

Psychiatric Issues

The rate of tobacco use is higher among psychiatrically impaired individuals as a whole when compared with a control population. It is also well known that psychotic patients who smoke tend to smoke heavily (23–25). Cessation of tobacco use is associated with, among other psychiatric conditions, an increased risk of relapse to depression, especially among women (26–28).

Withdrawal

Nicotine withdrawal is characterized by increased irritability, general restlessness, and craving for the drug. Evidence is also seen of cognitive problems during this time. Onset of symptoms begins within hours of discontinuing tobacco use and usually peaks within a few days. Patients complain of symptoms for several weeks after stopping nicotine. Weight gain and increased appetite are common during and after nicotine withdrawal (29,30).

Medical Consequences

The medical consequences of nicotine use are extremely well documented, and an exhaustive review is beyond the scope of this discussion. It is clear, however, that nicotine use results in problems in numerous organ systems. Among its cardiovascular effects are hypertension and increased risk of myocardial infarctions caused by vasospasm and an increase in thrombogenesis. A variety of cancers are increased in smokers, with the most obvious being lung and oropharyngeal cancer. The presence of nicotine and the particulate matter that occurs as a result of tobacco use worsens the course of all pulmonary diseases, including exacerbating asthma, causing emphysema, and increasing the risk of pneumonias and other upper airway infections.

ALCOHOL: BRIEF HISTORY

The history of alcohol is difficult to trace—more difficult than is that of the more straightforward nicotine. It is clear from pictures and writings that in 3200 BC the Sumerians enjoyed a beverage similar to beer. Wines too were recognized by about this time. Because of the spontaneous occurrence of fermentation, it is not possible to say with certainty where this ubiquitous substance originated (31).

Absorption and Elimination

Alcohol, C_2H_5OH, is a simple molecule with solubility in both lipid and water. It easily diffuses across membrane and enters the system quickly. The drug is distributed throughout the body and tissues, with extremely rapid uptake into brain. Alcohol (ethanol) has rapid and complete absorption in the gastrointestinal (GI) tract, especially the upper GI. Absorption is potentially dependent on how recently the individual has eaten, so that an empty stomach takes up alcohol rapidly, whereas some delay occurs after feeding. Because of this, the time to peak blood levels will range from about 30 to 90 minutes.

Of ethanol, 95% is metabolized by way of alcohol dehydrogenase. The 5% remaining is excreted unchanged, primarily through the lungs. Most metabolism occurs in the liver. Approximately 15%, however, occurs in the stomach by way of alcohol dehydrogenase located in the stomach lining. It is interesting to note that, given the same amount of ethanol by body weight, women demonstrate a higher level of blood alcohol than men. Women have about half the amount of alcohol dehydrogenase in their stomachs that men have, and are unable to metabolize ethanol as quickly.

Alcohol appears to facilitate the action of γ-aminobutyric acid (GABA), an inhibitory neurotransmitter, thus exerting an overall depression on CNS function.

Physiologic Response

The user of alcohol initially demonstrates increased respiration. With increasing levels of ethanol, however, the respiratory suppression characteristic of other depressants results in slowed respiration, the cause of death in overdoses. Other CNS depressants combined with alcohol cause a strongly additive effect. This combination can result in death at lower levels of either. A person ingesting alcohol experiences a warm, flushing sensation caused by dilation of blood vessels to the skin. As a result of this vasodilatation, it is possible for the individual who has ingested alcohol to freeze to death more quickly and after briefer exposure to the cold than would otherwise be the case. At low doses, alcohol has a protective effect on the heart. At high doses, however, the protective effect is lost and the individual is at increased risk of cardiomyopathy, among other cardiovascular problems. A confounding issue here, however, is what constitutes "high" and "low" doses. Great individual variation is seen, based on size, gender, and genetic influences, thus this information must be viewed with much caution.

Alcohol also acts to decrease the secretion of antidiuretic hormone. Thus, the frequent urination that drinkers experience is not simply caused by volume overload, but also by the fact that the body is not actively seeking to retain fluid as it would under normal circumstances. This fact has particular importance for the individual on some types of medications and those with underlying medical conditions where dehydration can place them at serious risk.

Behavioral effects of alcohol are unpredictable, depending, to some degree, on the individual and that person's expectations. At low doses, the user often feels a slight stimulation, with expansive mood and euphoria. With continued ingestion, however, the sedative effects predominate.

Pregnancy

Of the female population, 4% are alcohol-abusing or alcohol-dependent and the number appears to be rising among younger women. Women develop physical and cognitive problems associated with alcohol use after lower level consumption and after a briefer period of time than do men. Although various popular drugs of abuse have been suspected of causing fetal abnormalities, only alcohol is known unequivocally to be teratogenic. Alcohol freely crosses the placenta and the fetal blood–brain barrier so that fetal alcohol levels equal maternal levels. Deleterious effects of alcohol on the fetus have been recognized at least since Biblical times, as, for example, when an angel of God tells a woman that she has conceived and must now "drink no wine nor strong drink" (Judges 13:7). In 19th century Europe, concern was raised about the condition of offspring born to alcoholic women. It was not until 1969, however, that an accurate description was made of the effect of alcohol on the fetus. A constellation of physical and mental abnormalities occurs in the offspring of 30% to 50% of alcohol-dependent mothers, termed fetal alcohol syndrome (FAS) or alcohol-related neurodevelopmental disorder (32). Evidence suggests that the expression of FAS is related to peak alcohol levels. Thus, it may be that heavy binging of alcohol resulting in high peak levels produces the most serious effects on the fetus (33). Because it is not known what constitutes an acceptable level of alcohol exposure to the fetus, any amount of use of this drug should be discouraged in pregnancy. Studies have shown that cessation of alcohol during pregnancy is associated with a better fetal outcome and less severe sequelae. Thus, a woman should be encouraged to stop drinking regardless of what level of fetus gestation. Warren and Foudin (34), for the National Institute on Alcohol Abuse and Alcoholism, summarize a number of studies regarding risk factors for the development of FAS. They indicate that it is associated with older age, poorer socioeconomic status, ethnicity, genetic factors, maternal metabolism, among others, as well as peak alcohol levels (Table 4-1).

Medical Complications of Alcohol Abuse and Dependence

The medical consequences of alcohol misuse affect virtually every organ system. No effort is made here to supply an exhaustive review of the health consequences of alcohol use as they are well known and extensive. Some of the problems are related to nutritional deficiencies attendant on heavy alcohol ingestion (e.g., folic acid and thiamine deficiencies). Others are related to the direct toxic effect of the drug on specific organ systems. Most widely recognized are the effects of alcohol on the GI system. Liver damage, cirrhosis, liver failure, pancreatitis, gastritis, peptic ulcer disease, and esophageal and rectal varices are all common sequelae of heavy alcohol consumption. Neurologic sequelae, including brain damage in the form of the irreversible dementing condition Wernicke-Korsakov syndrome, as well as peripheral neuropathies are also well described. In addition, cardiomyopathy, hypertension, and bone marrow suppression with macrocytic anemia are frequent complications of alcohol dependence.

Withdrawal and Detoxification

Withdrawal from some substances of abuse constitutes little more than a nuisance and passing discomfort to the individual. Withdrawal from alcohol and other CNS depressants, however, poses the risk of seizure and even death. Alcohol withdrawal symptoms generally have their onset within 24 to 72 hours after cessa-

Table 4-1.   Fetal alcohol syndrome and alcohol-related effects (34)

Category I. FAS with confirmed maternal alcohol use: (use confirmed plus)
A. Characteristic pattern of facial anomalies, including short palpebral fissures, flattened midface and philtrum
B. Growth retardation
C. Neurodevelopmental abnormalities: can be hard or soft signs (e.g., small head at birth or abnormal sensorimotor development)

Category II. FAS without confirmed maternal alcohol use: (use not confirmed plus)
A–C above

Category III. Partial FAS with confirmed maternal alcohol use: (use confirmed plus)
A. Some facial patterns above plus *either B, C, or D below*
B. Growth retardation, as in category I
C. Neurodevelopmental abnormalities, as in category I
D. Other behavioral or cognitive abnormalities inconsistent with developmental level and without other obvious explanations

Category IV. Alcohol-related birth defects
A. Confirmed maternal alcohol use
B. One or more congenital malformations

Category V. Alcohol-related neurodevelopmental disorder
A. Confirmed maternal alcohol use
B. Neurodevelopmental abnormalities, as in category I *and/or*
C. Behavioral or cognitive deficits, as in category III

ARE, alcohol-related effects; FAS, fetal alcohol syndrome. (From Warren KR, Foudin LL. Alcohol related birth defects—the past, present, and future. *Alcohol Res Health* 2001;25(3):153–158)

tion of drinking; or, in the case of individuals who consistently maintains alcohol in their body (e.g., the individual who drinks daily throughout the day), once a significant decrease in alcohol level has occurred. The withdrawal syndrome can be preceded by the onset of seizure activity. If such occurs, it will usually be within the first 12 to 24 hours after last alcohol ingestion.

Alcohol withdrawal is characterized by autonomic arousal, which can be mediated through the GABA-ergic system. That is, alcohol ingestion causes an increase in GABA activity which, in turn, serves to have a tranquilizing effect on the CNS. When the alcohol effect is withdrawn, the inhibitory effect of GABA is likewise withdrawn, resulting in a sudden increase in CNS activity. Signs and symptoms of alcohol withdrawal include tremors and restlessness. The individual may experience shaking chills, but only a modest elevation in temperature. A rise of more than 2°F of temperature should prompt a search for another source to explain this finding. The patient will show a tachycardia and hypertension and can become delirious as well. The syndrome should have run its course completely by the end of about 7 days (Table 4-2).

Table 4-2. Overview: some medical consequences of alcohol abuse

System	Consequence
Gastrointestinal	Pancreatitis, liver disease; gastric, esophageal, or duodenal ulceration; esophageal or rectal varices
Cardiovascular	Cardiomyopathy, hypertension
Hematologic	Bone marrow suppression; macrocytic anemia; thrombocytopenia
Nutritional	Folic acid deficiency; thiamine deficiency; vitamins D/A/E/K deficiency
Neurologic	Peripheral neuropathies; Wernicke-Korsakov; Marchiafava-Bignami; cerebellar ataxia, and so forth

CANNABIS

The hemp plant, *Cannabis sativa,* has been valued for its many properties since ancient times. The usefulness of its fibers for making such things as nets and ropes was recognized as early as 10,000 BC in China. References to the psychoactive properties of cannabis, the product of its flowers, leaves, and resin, are found in literature from that same country by 2700 BC. In the first century AD, references to its medicinal and intoxicating effects appeared both in China and in the Middle East. It was not until the 19th century, however, that soldiers who had served in the Far East introduced the intoxicant to Europe (1,35).

Marijuana is a "dirty" drug, in which more than sixty cannabinoids are present. The most important psychoactive properties of cannabis come from the substance, δ-9 tetrahydrocannabinol (THC), which primarily is used by either ingesting or smoking the substance. THC is insoluble in water and must be extracted with alcohol in order to inject the drug, thus i.v. administration is a rarity. Although "marijuana" is the most commonly recognized name for THC-containing drugs, it is also present in other preparations with different percentages of THC (Table 4-3).

The effect of marijuana depends, in part, on the user's expectation and environment of use, in addition to possibly some genetically determined factors. Although listed as a narcotic, schedule I drug, marijuana is actually a sedative at low doses. At higher doses, it is capable of inducing hallucinations.

In one national study, more than a third of Americans admitted to having used marijuana at some time, whereas 13% were considered current users (36).

Absorption and Elimination

Highly fat-soluble, THC can cross the blood–brain barrier very quickly. Onset, intensity, and duration of effect are dependent on the route of administration. When the user inhales a single puff

Table 4-3. THC-containing preparations

Preparation	Source	THC (%)
Marijuana	Leaves	1–3
Sensemilla	Female flower	3–6
Ganja	Highly compressed female flower	4–8
Hashish	Plant tar	10–15
Hashish oil	Elixir of plant tar	20–60

THC, tetrahydrocannabinol.

of cannabis, THC finds its way to brain receptors within seconds, giving the user a very rapid onset of action. Peak level occurs within less than 30 minutes, although the most intense euphoria of the "high" lingers up to 4 hours longer.

Oral ingestion delivers a variable dose of THC to the brain, with absorption speed varying, depending on whether the individual has eaten, for example. Onset of action can take up to an hour and peak blood levels can be delayed for several hours when the user consumes THC this way. The high, however, will last up to 8 hours.

Because of its lipid solubility, THC is easily absorbed throughout the body and tissue. It is metabolized in the liver and excreted from the body in the urine (33%) and in the feces (66%). As the elimination half-life is 3 to 5 days, daily use of THC can result in accumulation of the drug in the body that will be metabolized out only after a prolonged period. Thus, in a habitual user, a toxicologic screen can stay positive for several weeks after the last use of the drug.

The exact manner in which THC affects the CNS is unclear. It does appear, however, that special receptors for cannabinoids exist in highest density in the cerebral cortex, especially the frontal areas, the basal ganglia, globus pallidus, and substantia nigra, cerebellum, and hippocampus. The brainstem lacks cannabinoid receptors, which may be the reason that THC is apparently not a lethal drug.

Physiologic Effects

The desired effect of THC is its ability to produce relaxation and euphoria. It has much more generalized physiologic effects as well, however. THC has a strong effect on the cardiovascular system. A transient increase in blood pressure may be seen in an inexperienced user, but the typical effect is of a lowering of the blood pressure because of vasodilation. This is accompanied by the anticipated compensatory increase in heart rate. The vasodilation is the cause of the familiar reddening of the conjunctivae characteristic of the user. It may also be the cause of decreased intraocular pressure that is exploited when glaucoma sufferers smoke the drug.

Central nervous system effects of THC vary with the surroundings, the expectation of the user, and with the dose delivered to the brain. Users report experiences ranging from mild euphoria to deep sleep producing intoxication, to hallucinations, panic, and psychosis. THC worsens psychomotor function. The user may appear clumsy and exhibit poor balance control. Under the influence of THC, the user displays significantly delayed reaction time; thus, driving performance, for example, is impaired.

Despite assertions by users of marijuana that THC enhances their sensitivity to others and to their surroundings, it is clear that this drug makes the intoxicated user less aware of auditory and visual stimuli. In addition, the user's attention span is decreased and the ability to perform tasks requiring concentration is reduced. Of greater concern is that acute THC intoxication seriously inhibits the user's ability to learn new material. Thus, the adolescent who chronically uses the drug will find it difficult to perform at an adequate level in school. It appears, however, that these effects are limited to the time of intoxication, and research has failed to demonstrate a long-term reduction in IQ of the user. It should be noted, however, that because of the long half-life and tissue accumulation of THC, the period of feeling intoxicated can outlast the period of obvious intoxication.

Considerations in Pregnancy

Research regarding outcome of offspring of mothers who use marijuana during gestation is made difficult by simultaneous use of other drugs, especially tobacco, with its known fetal effects. Currently, no good evidence indicates growth abnormalities in marijuana-exposed neonates, including significant changes in birthweight. Data are contradictory whether marijuana use during pregnancy causes an increase in the risk of SIDS (37–40).

Medical Consequences

Studies show that both marijuana and cigarettes have many of the same carcinogens. Despite this, no clear evidence shows that cannabis causes cancer. Concern exists, however, that future findings may show that cannabis use, as with tobacco, increases the likelihood of cancer, because the population of marijuana users is only now entering the cancer age. Also conflicting data exist whether this drug causes significant pulmonary changes, although given the mechanism of damage caused by nicotine, it would seem likely.

Concerns have been raised that THC may exert a negative effect on the immune system and also cause a decrease in production of sex hormones. These questions are still unanswered by controlled research, which has produced variable results.

Withdrawal

Withdrawal from cannabis is not listed as a syndrome in the *Diagnostic and Statistical Manual of Mental Disorders*-IV and is not clinically significant. Nevertheless, long-time users complain of a number of symptoms, including sleep and appetite disturbances, anxiety, nausea, and perhaps increased aggression (41). It appears that the peak symptoms occur within 3 to 5 days of cessation of marijuana use, but can last for several weeks thereafter (Table 4-3).

STIMULANTS

The stimulant drugs include a variety of substances, both naturally occurring and synthetic. The general effects are the same and cocaine, the original, naturally occurring psychostimulant, is discussed as the prototype.

Cocaine is the product of the leaves of the coca plant, *Erythroxylon coca,* primarily harvested in South America, in Bolivia, Peru, and Columbia. The Andean Indians, who chewed the leaves of the coca plant, first exploited its psychoactive properties. Mixed with ashes from the fire, coca decreased the need for food and increased the user's energy level (1). Cocaine's usefulness as an anesthetic agent was demonstrated in the 1880s when it was used for performing ophthalmological surgery. Its intoxicant effects were also discovered at about the same time and the drug was used widely by medical professionals, including Sigmund Freud, and in the popular literature (e.g., by Sherlock Holmes) (42,43).

Absorption and Elimination

Depending on how it is prepared, cocaine can be smoked, injected, or snorted. In its least prepared form, cocaine exists as cocaine hydrochloride, and is typically used intranasally or intravenously. Cocaine in this form is commonly adulterated or "cut" with similar appearing substances that mimic some of its effects (e.g., mannitol, lactose).

Cocaine freebase is a smokeable form in which a strong base is added to the drug and heated. The precipitate, which has a lower melting point, is smoked either alone or combined in a tobacco cigarette. The process of "freebasing" often involves the use of highly volatile substances (e.g., ether) and injuries have occurred when that substance was exposed to heat and exploded.

A third popular form of cocaine is that of so called "crack" or "rock" cocaine. It too has a lower melting point than cocaine hydrochloride, and can be smoked, allowing for very rapid delivery to the brain via the massive absorptive surface of the lungs. "Crack" is made by first combining the drug with a strong base, and then dissolving, heating, and leaving it to dry into a crystalline form. "Crack" derives its name from the sharp snapping sound heard when the mixture is prepared. Although cocaine in all its forms causes tolerance and dependence, a more rapid advancement to compulsive use occurs with smoking "crack" or "freebase" because of the extremely rapid delivery of high doses of the drug to the brain.

Depending on the route of administration, the onset of action of cocaine can appear to be nearly instantaneous, with the most intense feeling subsiding within 15 to 30 minutes with crack or freebase, after which the user feels impelled to use again. Most of the effect will be completely over by the end of 2 hours. One reviewer suggests that intranasal administration of the drug results in a less-intense, but more prolonged effect of cocaine because of vasoconstriction (44).

Physiologic Response

The desired effect of cocaine is to increase the user's energy and decrease his or her need for food and sleep. In the new user, these effects are accompanied by increased sexual appetite, although this effect diminishes greatly over time. As cocaine exerts its effects on the sympathetic nervous system, some of its effects on the user are predictable. An individual using cocaine experiences a rapid and profound increase in heart rate and blood pressure. The user's pupils dilate, body temperature increases, bowels move, and restlessness sets in.

Medical Consequences

The combination of the hypertensive and tachycardic effects of cocaine has been known to result in angina, myocardial and other types of organ infarctions, strokes, and seizures. Cardiac dysrhythmias have been known to occur as well.

Psychiatric Consequences

Along with an increase in activity, cocaine users may display increased aggression. Suspiciousness and paranoia are common features of the chronic cocaine user as well (45,46). The combination of these responses obviously can lead to a dangerous situation and violence can occur. Cocaine use alone can result in a picture of paranoid psychosis that can mimic the symptoms of schizophrenia, although in the individual who does not have an underlying psychotic process, it tends to be time limited (47,48). In addition, it can worsen psychotic symptoms in individuals already predisposed to such. The risk of suicide is greatly increased in the context of cocaine use and in the immediate period after cocaine use. Thus, threats or suicidal ideation during this period should not be taken lightly (49–52).

Pregnancy

Because of the dramatic rise in the numbers of cocaine-exposed neonates born in the last decade and a half, much attention has focused on the effect of this drug on the pregnant mother and her offspring. Cocaine crosses the placenta quickly and is metabolized slowly by the fetus, thus exposing it to the drug for prolonged periods of time. Cocaine can have a profound effect on the pregnant uterus and fetus. Its use is associated with an increased risk of placental abruption and premature rupture of the membranes, with resultant fetal oxygen deprivation (53). It appears that cocaine use increases the risk of spontaneous abortion as well (15). In addition, the rise in blood pressure that the mother experiences during cocaine use can also occur in the fetus, increasing the risk of intracerebral bleed in both mother and fetus.

Babies born to cocaine-dependent mothers tend to suffer from intrauterine growth retardation and to have a smaller occipitofrontal measurement and length, especially when the drug is used during the last trimester (15).

No consensus is found on the long-term effects of cocaine on the neonate. Some evidence indicates difficulties in attention and behavior may occur among children exposed to cocaine *in utero* whose severity appears in a dose-dependent fashion. Evidence is seen of motor changes among cocaine-exposed toddlers as well (54–58).

Withdrawal

Withdrawal from cocaine is characterized by lethargy and sleepfulness, but without restful sleep and with depression. Suicide is a considerable danger at this time, and the individual user may require hospitalization for safety. The most severe of these symptoms usually resolve in 2 or 3 days. In the nonsuicidal user, cocaine withdrawal is not a life-threatening situation (Table 4-4).

OPIOIDS

The opioid family of drugs encompasses a number of substances both naturally occurring and synthetic, with the most widely rec-

Table 4-4. Cocaine preparations

	Preparation	Route of Administration
Cocaine hydrochloride powder	Mixed with a sugar (e.g., mannitol or lactose)	Intravenous or intranasal
Freebase cocaine	Addition of a base (e.g., NH_3) to a liquid solution of cocaine; heated and the precipitate collected	Smoked
Crack cocaine	Mixed with baking soda, formed into a solution; heated and permitted to dry into a crystalline form	Smoked

ognized opioids of abuse being heroin and morphine. For a list of examples of other opioids, see Table 4-5. Naturally occurring members of the opioid class are derived from opium, the product of the opium poppy, *Papaver somniferum.* The benefits of opium for the treatment of diarrhea, for pain relief, and for sleep have been well described for more than 5,000 years. It appears that the addictive properties of the poppy were also recognized, as references warning against the plant's use can be found in the third century BC (59). All opioid narcotics act as CNS depressants and can cause respiratory depression and death at high doses. The raw form of the opium poppy was smoked for centuries, until the early 1800s when a much purer drug was extracted, and morphine, named for the god Morpheus, emphasizing its dream-inducing capability, was introduced.

Absorption and Elimination

It is difficult to lump the opioids together, as different preparations have been purposely developed for absorption from different sites. Morphine, however, is incompletely absorbed from the GI

Table 4-5. Examples of opioid preparations

Generic Name	Example	Half-life (hr)
Codeine	Codeine	3–4
Fentanyl	Actiq	1–6
Hydrocodone	Vicodin	3–4.5
Hydromorphone	Dilaudid	2–4
Methadone	Dolophine	15–30
Morphine	Roxanol	2–4
Oxycodone	OxyContin	3–4
Propoxyphene	Darvon	3–15

tract and is better absorbed intravenously. Most of its metabolism is in the liver.

Physiologic Response

The initial response typically elicited to opioid administration is that of nausea and vomiting caused by a direct effect on the area postrema. The committed user, however, adapts to the emetic effect and this response disappears. Opioid use, in direct contrast to cocaine use, results in pinpoint pupils, thus the caricature of the addict with the ever present "shades." The user will feel euphoric, although sedated; may doze, but is easily roused. Onset of action is typically seconds to minutes, depending on the route of administration.

Medical Consequences of Heroin Use

Compared with other drugs of abuse, the effect of heroin and other opioids on the body are really mild and center almost entirely on the route of administration and the presence of contaminants in street drugs. Opioids themselves cause constipation, which if severe enough can result in paralysis of the gut. Death from opioid overdose is the result of respiratory depression and the individual demonstrates signs of pulmonary edema.

Psychiatric

Opioid use does not appear to induce psychiatric symptoms of its own, although, as will be seen in subsequent chapters, many psychiatric conditions are found among opioid users.

Pregnancy

Offspring of opioid-dependent women who continue to use heroin throughout pregnancy are at a significantly increased risk of neonatal mortality (60). They tend to be smaller in weight and shorter, with a smaller occipitofrontal circumference as well (61). In addition, although seizure activity is uncommon in adults withdrawing from opioids alone, it is an occurrence that must be guarded against in the neonate (62). It is important to note that heroin babies whose mothers are maintained on methadone are larger, healthier, and at reduced risk of perinatal difficulties compared with babies whose mothers are on heroin alone and babies whose mothers are on methadone but continue to use heroin as well (63).

Withdrawal

In an otherwise healthy individual, opioid withdrawal is not typically a life-threatening experience, although it is extremely uncomfortable. Onset of withdrawal will occur after approximately one half-life of the drug on which the patient is dependent. Thus, a heroin-dependent patient can anticipate beginning to experience some mild withdrawal symptoms after 6 hours of the last use of the drug. If methadone is the drug the patient uses, withdrawal symptoms can be expected after approximately 24 hours. Withdrawal will advance to lacrimation, rhinorrhea, yawning, piloerection, nausea, vomiting, diarrhea, muscle cramps, and twitching. It is important to note that, unlike with other opiates, seizure activity is a possibility in meperidine withdrawal. Table 4-6 provides a summary of the discussion above.

Table 4-6. Review: action of drugs of abuse

Substance	Action	Physiologic Response	Withdrawal	Medical Considerations	Issues with Pregnancy
Cocaine	Stimulant	↑BP, ↑HR, ↑Temp. ↑Energy, ↑Paranoia ↓Fatigue, ↓Appetite Move bowels or urinate	Lethargy Fatigue Depression (may be life-threatening)	Stroke; cardiovascular collapse; myocardial and other organ infarction; paranoia; violence; severe depression; suicide	Risk of infarcts to fetal organs; placental abruptions
Ethanol	Sedative	Sedation ↓Respiration, CNS depression, coma, death	↑BP, ↑HR, ↑Temp Nausea, vomiting, diarrhea Seizures, delirium, death	Virtually every organ system affected: cardiomyopathy, liver disease, esophageal and rectal varices, to name a few	Fetal alcohol syndrome Multiple alcohol effects

Continued

Table 4-6. *Continued*

Substance	Action	Physiologic Response	Withdrawal	Medical Considerations	Issues with Pregnancy
Heroin (other opioids)	Sedative, euphoriant	Nausea, pin-point pupils, constipation, analgesia	Nausea, vomiting, diarrhea, piloerection, lacrimation, rhinorrhea, yawning	Depends upon route of administration and preference of contaminants	Lower birth weight, length, head circumference
Cannabis (Delta-9, tetrahydrocannabinol)		↓BP, ↑HR, ↓intraocular pressure, conjunctival injection	↑Irritability Sleep disturbance ?Nausea ?Vomiting	Euphoriant, may cause hallucinations	Unknown
Nicotine	Stimulant	Norepinephrine release, ↑HR, ↑BP	↑Irritability, weight gain. May last for weeks	Delayed wound healing, enlargement of heart, ↑risk of heart attack	Increase risk of spontaneous abortion, decreased fetal length/weight. Excreted in breast milk. Consequences unknown; latter are unknown. Increased risk of SIDS.

BP, blood pressure; CNS, central nervous system; HR, heart rate; SIDS, sudden infant death syndrome; Temp, temperature.

REFERENCES

1. Rudgley R. *The encyclopedia of psychoactive substances.* New York: St. Martin's Press, 1999.
2. Doll R, Peto R, Wheatley K, et al. Mortality in relation to smoking: forty years' observation on male British doctors. *BMJ* 1994;309 (6959):901–911.
3. Cocores J. Nicotine dependence: diagnosis and treatment. *Psychiatr Clin North Am* 1993;16:49.
4. Breslau N, Johnson EO, Hiripi E, et al. Nicotine dependence in the United States: prevalence, trends, and smoking persistence. *Arch Gen Psychiatry* 2001;58(9):810–816.
5. Studies Substance Abuse and Mental Health Service Administration. *Preliminary results from the 1997 National Household Survey.* Rockville, MD: National Institute of Health, 1998.
6. Peto R, Lopez AD, Boreham J, et al. Mortality from tobacco in developed countries: indirect estimation from national vital statistics. *Lancet* 1992;339:1268–1278.
7. Krueger JK, Rohrich RJ. Clearing the smoke: the scientific rationale for tobacco abstention with plastic surgery. *Plast Reconstr Surg* 2001;108(4):1063–1073.
8. Benowitz NL, Jacob PI. Individual differences in nicotine kinetics and metabolism in humans. In: Lee TNH, ed. *Molecular approaches to drug abuse research. III: Recent advances and emerging strategies,* Vol. 161. Rockville MD: US Department of Health and Human Services, 1996:48–64.
9. Ernst M, Heishman SJ, Spurgeon L, et al. Smoking history and nicotine effects on cognitive performance. *Neuropsychopharmacology* 2001;25(3):313–319.
10. Ernst M, Matochik JA, Heishman SJ, et al. Effect of nicotine on brain activation during performance of a working memory task. *Proc Natl Acad Sci USA* 2001;98(8):4728–4733.
11. Bell SL, Taylor RC, Singleton EG, et al. Smoking after nicotine deprivation enhances cognitive performance and decreases tobacco craving in drug users. *Nicotine Tob Res* 1999;1(1):45–52.
12. Mancuso G, Warburton DM, Melen M, et al. Selective effects of nicotine on attentional processes. *Psychopharmacology* 1999; 146(2):199–204.
13. Seidl R, Tiefenthaler M, Hauser E, et al. Effects of transdermal nicotine on cognitive performance in Down's syndrome. *Lancet* 2000;356(9239):1409–1410.
14. Founds J, Stapleton J, Swettenham J, et al. Cognitive performance effects of subcutaneous nicotine in smokers and never smokers. *Psychopharmacology* 1996;127(1):31–38.
15. Ness RBG, Hirschinger JA, Markovic N, et al. Cocaine and tobacco use and the risk of spontaneous abortion. *N Engl J Med* 1999; 340(5):333–339.
16. Shiverick KT, Salafia C. Cigarette smoking and pregnancy. I: Ovarian, uterine, and placental effects. *Placenta* 1999;20(4):265–272.
17. Economides D, Braithwaite J. Smoking, pregnancy and the fetus. *J R Soc Health* 1994;114(4):198–201.
18. Cornelius M, Taylor P, Geva D, et al. Prenatal tobacco and marijuana use among adolescents: effects on offspring gestational age, growth, and morphology. *Pediatrics* 1995;95(5):738–743.
19. Amir LH. Maternal smoking and reduced duration of breastfeeding: a review of possible mechanisms. *Early Hum Dev* 2001; 64(1):45–67.

20. Schwartz-Bickenback D, Schulte-Hobein B, Abt S, et al. Smoking and passive smoking during pregnancy and early infancy: effects on birth weight, lactation period, and cotinine concentrations in mother's milk and infant's urine. *Toxicol Lett* 1987;35(1): 73–81.

21. Wisborg K, Kesmodel U, Henriksen TB, et al. A prospective study of smoking during pregnancy and SIDS. *Arch Dis Child* 2000; 83(3):203–206.

22. Pollack HA. Sudden infant death syndrome, maternal smoking during pregnancy, and the cost effectiveness of smoking cessation intervention. *Am J Public Health* 2001;91(3):432–436.

23. Dalack GW, Healy DJ, Meador-Woodruff JH. Nicotine dependence in schizophrenia: clinical phenomena and laboratory findings. *Am J Psychiatry* 1998;155(11):1490–1501.

24. Itkin O, Nemets B, Einat H. Smoking habits in bipolar and schizophrenic outpatients in southern Israel. *J Clin Psychiatry* 2001; 62(4):269–272.

25. Kelly C, McCreadie RG. Smoking habits, current symptoms, and premorbid characteristics of schizophrenic patients in Nithsdale, Scotland. *Am J Psychiatry* 1999;156(11):1751–1757.

26. Glassman AH. Cigarette smoking: implications for psychiatric illness. *Am J Psychiatry* 1993;150(4):546–553.

27. Covey LSG, Alexander H, Stetner F. Major depression following smoking cessation. *Am J Psychiatry* 1997;154:263–265.

28. Quattrocki E, Baird A, Yurgelun-Todd D. Biological aspects of the link between smoking and depression. *Harv Rev Psychiatry* 2000; 83:99–110.

29. Hughes JR, Gust SW, Skoog Kea. Symptoms of tobacco withdrawal. *Arch Gen Psychiatry* 1991;48:52–59.

30. Hughes JR, Feiester S, Goldstein Mea. Practice guidelines for the treatment of patients with nicotine dependence. *Am J Psychiatry* 1996;153(Suppl):1–29.

31. Rudgley R. *Essential substances: a cultural history of intoxicants in society.* New York: Kodansha International, 1993.

32. Jones KL, Smith DW. Recognition of the fetal alcohol syndrome in early infancy. *Lancet* 1973;2:999–1001.

33. Chen W-JA, Maier SE, West JR. Toxic effects of ethanol on the fetal brain. In: Deitrich RA, Erwin VG, eds. *Pharmacological effects of ethanol on the nervous system.* Boca Raton, FL: CRC Press, 1996:343–361.

34. Warren KR, Foudin LL. Alcohol related birth defects—the past, present, and future. *Alcohol Res Health* 2001;25(3):153–158.

35. Iverson LL. *The science of marijuana.* New York: Oxford University Press, 2000.

36. Infofax N. *Marijuana.* Rockville, MD: National Institute on Drug Abuse, 2001:1–6.

37. English DR, Hulse GK, Milne E, et al. Maternal cannabis use and birth weight: a meta-analysis. *Addiction* 1997;92(11):1553–1560.

38. Fried PA, Watkinson B, Gray R. Growth from birth to early adolescence in offspring prenatally exposed to cigarettes and marijuana. *Neurotoxicol Teratol* 1999;21(5):513–525.

39. Ostrea EM, Ostrea AR, Simpson PM. Mortality within the first two years in infants exposed to cocaine, opiate, or cannabinoid during gestation. *Pediatrics* 1997;100(1):79–83.

40. Scragg RK, Mitchell EA, Ford RP, et al. Maternal cannabis use in the sudden death syndrome. *Acta Paediatrica* 2001;90(1):57–60.
41. Kouri EM, Pope HGJ Jr., Lukas SE. Changes in aggressive behavior during withdrawal from long term marijuana use. *Psychopharmacology* 1999;143(3):302–308.
42. Freud S. *The cocaine papers.* New York: Meridian Books, 1974.
43. Doyle SAC. *The complete Sherlock Holmes: all four novels and 56 short stories.* US, Bantam Classic and Loveswept, 1998.
44. Schuckit MA. *Drug and alcohol abuse: a clinical guide to diagnosis and treatment.* New York: Kluwer Academic/Plenum Publishers, 2000.
45. Sherer MA, Kumor KM, Cone EJ, et al. Suspiciousness induced by four-hour intravenous infusions of cocaine: preliminary findings. *Arch Gen Psychiatry* 1989;46(12):1152.
46. Williamson S, Gossop M, Powis B, et al. Adverse effects of stimulant drugs in a community sample of drug users. *Drug Alcohol Depend* 1997;44(2–3):87–94.
47. Satel SL, Seibyl JP, Charney DS. Prolonged cocaine psychosis implies underlying major psychopathology. *J Clin Psychiatry* 1991;52(8):349–350.
48. Harris D, Batki SL. Stimulant psychosis: symptom profile and acute clinical course. *Am J Addict* 2000;9(1):28–37.
49. Marzuk PM, Tardiff K, Leon AC, et al. Prevalence of cocaine use among residents of New York City who committed suicide during a one year period. *Am J Psychiatry* 1992;149(3):371–375.
50. Dhossche DM, Rich CL, Ghani SO, et al. Patterns of psychoactive substance detection from routine toxicology of suicides in Mobile Alabama between 1990 and 1998. *J Affect Disord* 2001;64(2–3):167–174.
51. Salloum IM, Daley DC, Cornelius JR, et al. Disproportionate lethality in psychiatric patients with concurrent alcohol and cocaine abuse. *Am J Psychiatry* 1996;153(7):953–955.
52. Petronis KR, Samuels JF, Moscicki EK, et al. An epidemiologic investigation of potential risk factors for suicide attempts. *Soc Psychiatry Psychiatr Epidemiol* 1990;25(4):193–199.
53. Shiono PH, Klebanoff MA, Nugent RP, et al. The impact of cocaine and marijuana use on low birth weight and preterm birth: a multicenter study. *Am J Obstet Gynecol* 1995;172(1 pt 1):19–27.
54. Singer LT, Arendt R, Minnes S, et al. Neurobehavioral outcomes of cocaine-exposed infants. *Neurotoxicol Teratol* 2000;22(5):653–666.
55. Singer LT, Arendt R, Minnes S, et al. Cognitive and motor outcomes of cocaine-exposed infants. *JAMA* 2002;287(15):1952–1960.
56. Chavkin W. Cocaine and pregnancy—time to look at the evidence. *JAMA* 2001;285(12):1626–1628.
57. Frank DA, Augustyn M, Knight WG, et al. Growth, development, and behavior in early childhood following prenatal cocaine exposure. *JAMA* 2001;285(12):1613–1625.
58. Hurt H, Malmud E, Betancourt LM, et al. A prospective comparison of developmental outcome of children with in utero cocaine exposure and controls using the Battelle Developmental Inventory. *J Dev Behav Pediatr* 2001;22(1):27–34
59. Ashley R. *Heroin: the myths and the facts.* New York: St. Martin's Press, 1972.

60. Hulse GK, Milne E, English DR, et al. Assessing the relationship between maternal opiate use and neonatal mortality. *Addiction* 1998;93(7):1033–1042.
61. Hulse GK, Milne E, English DR, et al. The relationship between maternal use of heroin and methadone and infant birth weight. *Addiction* 1997;93(11):1571–1579.
62. Herzlinger RA, Kandall SR, Vaughan HGJ. Neonatal seizures associated with narcotic withdrawal. *J Pediatr* 1977;91(4):638–641.
63. Stimmel B. Fetal outcome in narcotic-dependent women: the importance of the type of maternal narcotic used. *Am J Drug Alcohol Abuse* 1982;9(4):383–395.

5

Withdrawal

1. Typically, withdrawal from a substance is like the opposite of intoxication
2. Alcohol
   a. Withdrawal can be life-threatening
   b. Depending on the individual, can be conducted as an inpatient or outpatient
   c. Parameters given for deciding on inpatient versus outpatient detoxification are given
   d. Signs and symptoms
      i. Onset: 24 to 72 hours
      ii. Over: 5 to 7 days
      iii. Autonomic arousal
      iv. Seizures can occur typically within first 12 to 48 hours
      v. Temperature greater than 100.5°F should signal search for cause of fever other than withdrawal
   e. Detoxification should occur during pregnancy because of risks of ethanol to fetus
3. Cocaine withdrawal
   a. Hallmark: sleep disturbance and irritability
   b. Early period after cocaine withdrawal can be punctuated by suicidal depression: protected environment indicated if this occurs
   c. Medication not essential but can be given for the symptoms: recommendation for possible symptomatic treatment given
4. Opioid withdrawal
   a. Withdrawal seldom life-threatening: dehydration with electrolyte imbalance a possibility
   b. Signs and symptoms
      i. Onset dependent on specific opioid: heroin less than 24 hours
      ii. Rhinorrhea, lacrimation, muscles twitching, gooseflesh, nausea, vomiting, diarrhea
      iii. With heroin withdrawal is over within 5 to 6 days
      iv. Inpatient treatment rarely necessary
      v. Detoxification with tramadol a possibility
      vi. Pregnancy: contraindication to detoxification

Withdrawal from a substance typically is similar to the opposite of intoxication from that substance. Knowing what the effect of a drug is, it is possible to predict what withdrawal from that drug will be like. Thus, if a drug's primary effect is one of stimulation, withdrawal will be characterized by low energy and a need for sleep. If the effect is one of sedation, wakefulness and irritability will likely be the symptoms of withdrawal. Keeping in mind that use and withdrawal have opposite effects makes it easier to predict what a patient may experience at a given time.

ALCOHOL

Table 5-1 lists the signs and symptoms of alcohol withdrawal. Various schemes have been developed over the years for treating alcohol withdrawal. In some circumstances, clinicians have applied ethanol drips—administrating ethanol intravenously (i.v.) and titrating this downward to prevent the emergence of withdrawal

Table 5-1. **Signs and symptoms of alcohol withdrawal**

Increased heart rate	Increased respiratory rate
Slight increase in body temperature (<101°F)	+/– Seizure activity
Plethora	Nausea
Vomiting	Diarrhea
+/– Disorientation	+/– Auditory and visual hallucinations

symptoms. Although such will work for this purpose, its drawbacks are enormous: including difficulty titrating the dose, interaction with other drugs, and hepatotoxicity. In the United States, barbiturates and benzodiazepines (1) are the most widely used medications for achieving detoxification from alcohol. The low risk-to-benefit ratio (therapeutic index) of barbiturates, especially in combination with alcohol and the lack of systematic data to support their use, make them the less desirable of the approaches (2).

Although the most serious form of alcohol withdrawal, delirium tremens (DTs) can be life-threatening, uncomplicated alcohol withdrawal may not require hospitalization to complete the process of detoxification. Alcohol withdrawal occurs on a continuum ranging from tremors and headache to frank DTs, characterized by vivid auditory and visual hallucinations and autonomic instability. DTs occur in 5% to 10% of alcohol-dependent individuals, and the condition is more likely to occur in individuals with other underlying medical and central nervous system conditions (3). In an otherwise healthy individual with no prior history of DTs or withdrawal seizures, withdrawal can be completed in an outpatient environment if the patient has the ability to follow directions and comprehend risks and has someone to help and support them. In this situation, daily visits are necessary to monitor blood pressure, heart rate, sensorium, and temperature and receive medications.

It is recommended that the clinician become familiar and comfortable with one or two ways of approaching alcohol withdrawal. Most clinicians in the United States use either a long- or a short-acting benzodiazepine for this purpose. Each way is effective and has its own relative benefits and drawbacks (3). Withdrawal with chlordiazepoxide, for example, has the advantage or requiring less frequent administration. It has the drawbacks, however, of being metabolized in the liver and of having active metabolites. In the individual with impaired liver function, this can mean prolonged action of the basic drug as well as accumulation of metabolites, which can result in sudden sedation after several days of administration. The short-acting agent, lorazepam, although metabolized in the liver, has no active metabolites, thus making drug accumulation impossible. However, its shorter half-life requires more frequent administration.

Signs and Symptoms of Alcohol Withdrawal

Onset of alcohol withdrawal occurs from 12 to 72 hours of the time that the individual's blood alcohol level drops. It is extremely

Table 5-2. Inpatient vs. outpatient alcohol detoxification: issues in determining whether inpatient or outpatient alcohol detoxification is preferred

Inability to arrive at clinic on a daily basis	In-patient indicated
History of delirium tremens or withdrawal seizures	Contraindication to outpatient detox: recurrence likely
Incapable of informed consent	Protective environment indicated
Suicidal or homicidal	Protective environment indicated
Able or willing to follow recommended treatment	Protective environment indicated if unable
Comorbid medical conditions	Unstable diabetes, hypertension, pregnancy, for example, all relatively strong contraindications to outpatient detox
Supportive other to assist	Not essential but advisable for outpatient detoxification

important to note that this does not mean that the individual's alcohol level must be zero to have withdrawal occur. It is possible that some patients are permitted to go into withdrawal because of the mistaken notion that such will not occur as long as alcohol remains in the patient's body. The important issue is that the level has dropped to a point that the central nervous system becomes aroused. If the patient is one who drinks throughout the day, thus consistently having an alcohol level, withdrawal seizures could occur and the patient still have a significant blood alcohol level. The symptoms will be seen to peak by 3 days and generally be over by 5 to 7 days. If the patient begins to display a delirium only after 7 days of alcohol cessation, the clinician should look for a cause other than alcohol withdrawal, as this is well outside the anticipated time course for onset of withdrawal symptoms. See Table 5-2 and Figure 5-1 for issues to consider when determining the correct venue for detoxification and a decision tree for this purpose.

CASE 5-1

Jack S., 39 years of age, was arrested at 11:30 on Saturday night for driving while intoxicated. Around noon on Sunday, he was rushed to the hospital after being found on the floor of his cell, shaking, writhing, and not responding to efforts to calm him. The episode was over by the time he arrived at the hospital. However, on the basis of the information received and the fact that Jack was unable to state whether or not he had ever had a seizure disorder, the doctors gave him a loading dose of phenytoin and he was returned to jail. Sometime before dawn the next morning, Jack was returned to the hospital strapped to a stretcher. He was combative, frightened, and screaming that

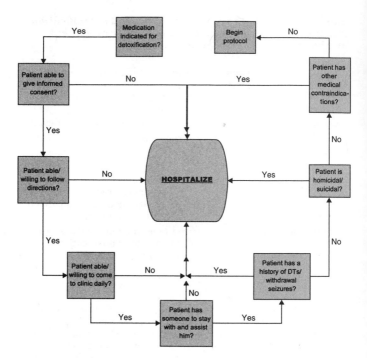

Figure 5-1.

there were skeletons threatening him. His blood pressure was elevated at 185/120, his pulse rate was 126. His body temperature was not adequately recorded in the emergency room. With difficulty, because of the patient's total lack of cooperation, an i.v. line was inserted; the patient received thiamine, a shot of vitamin K, and lorazepam (i.v.) was started before admission to the hospital.

This case is typical of the time course of onset of DTs and is a common scenario in jail facilities dealing with this population.

Pregnancy

Withdrawal during pregnancy is critical. Alcohol, of all the substances of abuse is the one known, true teratogen. As noted in Chapter 4, it is not known what level of alcohol is safe or at what point in gestation exposure to alcohol ceases to make a difference to the fetus. Animal studies show that ethanol exposure causes differential effects in the fetus throughout gestation even into the third trimester. This implies that stopping alcohol use should be encouraged regardless of where a woman is in her pregnancy (4). The question then becomes one of how to detoxify a woman from alcohol. This is best done in an inpatient setting with the assistance and close monitoring of a skilled obstetric team. The exact regimen to follow will be determined by the team's comfort with the use of benzodiazepines and barbiturates, the point in gestation, and the patient's specific response to each intervention. It cannot be over emphasized, however, that observation and medication for withdrawal must be given as needed.

Inpatient or Outpatient?

Nothing is absolute, but some guidelines to follow in determining the right placement for a given patient are discussed below.

Ability to Attend Clinic

Clearly, many fine plans have failed because the patient was unable to comply with the plan devised.

History of DTs and Withdrawal Seizures

A history of DTs and withdrawal seizures should be considered an absolute contraindication to attempt outpatient detoxification. A phenomenon known as "kindling" occurs. This phenomenon predicts that each time a person goes through withdrawal, the nervous system becomes more sensitized. Once the individual has had withdrawal seizures or DTs, the nervous system is so sensitive that each time it goes through any withdrawal, it takes less to "spark" new episodes of DTs and seizures. Just as kindling makes fires easier to ignite, less alcohol and briefer episodes of drinking are necessary to cause such patients to proceed to withdrawal seizures and DTs with successive episodes of withdrawal. Thus, monitoring is necessary. It should be noted, however, that many patients believe that any withdrawal symptoms from alcohol including mild shakes and tremors constitute "DTs," although clearly such is not the case. Rather than asking patients if they have had "DT," the clinician should ask specifically about auditory and visual hallucinations, how ill the individual was, whether hospitalized, what the patient remembers about the episode, and what treatment was rendered before deciding that the individual truly had "DTs."

In regard to seizure activity, once withdrawal seizures have occurred the patient is increasingly likely to have such again for each withdrawal. After someone has had a seizure, further such activity can be reduced by adding a benzodiazepine (e.g., lorazepam), although they cannot always be prevented (5). In addition, no evidence indicates that adding an agent such as phenytoin prophylactically will prevent the emergence of seizures (6). Thus, a history of either condition—DTs or withdrawal seizures—should signal the need for an inpatient admission.

Capacity for Informed Consent

It is essential to determine that the individual is capable of comprehending the regimen to follow and of giving truly informed consent. Although such issues are discussed in the specific chapters, an example might be an acutely psychotic man who believes alternately that he should take all his medication at one time to purge the alcohol and be relieved of his symptoms forever and that he should throw away all the pills because the voices told him whisky would make him free. Such an individual could not logically be expected to follow an outpatient detoxification regimen reliably. Likewise, someone who is in the throes of early dementia would not be a good candidate for outpatient, unmonitored withdrawal. In addition, daily monitoring is strongly advised, as the individual's condition can change. The person who begins an outpatient detoxification regimen on day 1, but is tachycardic, hypertensive, and seeing skeletons threatening him or her on day 2 can no longer be said to be a candidate for continued outpatient medication.

Suicidal or Homicidal?

A recurring theme throughout this text will be that individuals with dual diagnoses are the highest risk of all individuals for self-harm and increased risk of aggression. As is always the case, active suicidal ideation with a plan should be a signal for inpatient admission. Further, this supports daily visits for reassessment of the patient's mental status plan as well as prescription of medications. In general, benzodiazepines are safe medications, even in high doses. A week's worth of such medications mixed with a couple of fifths of whiskey, however, may not be.

Medical Conditions

A variety of conditions may make outpatient detoxification, inadvisable and require closer monitoring in a hospital environment. Conditions such as diabetes, especially insulin-dependent diabetes; unstable hypertension; a history of myocardial infarction or stroke, and unstable angina; pregnancy where monitoring of the fetal response is desirable; and any other condition of concern to the clinician are reasons to require inpatient rather than outpatient detoxification from alcohol.

Supportive Other

Although not an absolute requirement, a supportive other is highly desirable, and may have legal as well as medical ramifications. Benzodiazepine labeling contains a caveat against driving and operating heavy machinery. Thus, a problem may exist if a patient is driving to the office to get medications while under the influence of a benzodiazepine. In addition, because the patient can become more ill than anticipated, someone should be observing the patient and be able to bring him to the hospital for rehydration or admission, if necessary.

CASE 5-2

Bill T., 32 years of age, had a drinking problem and knew it. Because of his chronic absenteeism, he had lost his job and, as a result, his insurance. Bill and his wife had both witnessed him trying to stop drinking on his own many times. Each time, he had resumed, often with her blessings, because he had seemed so sick when he did not drink. When he tried to stop his hands shook. The dry heaves gave way to violent fits of vomiting, and his bloodshot eyes frightened her. They both knew that just a drink or two would take the symptoms away. Now, however, they were asking for help. If they could get some medication to get him through the worst part, they would come to the detoxifi-

*cation center every day and continue together in the program.
Bill did not have any particular medical problems—yet—that
he knew of. His blood pressure, 20 hours after his last drink
was 155/110 and his pulse 110. Thirty minutes after taking
lorazepam (1 mg), his blood pressure was 125/94 and his pulse
88. He felt better than he had felt all day. With prescriptions in
hand, Bill and his wife left, promising to return in 24 hours.*

Once the determination is made whether outpatient or inpatient
admission is necessary, the issue of what to do in terms of medication regimens remains. Ample evidence suggests that administration of medication only as symptoms arise is associated with shorter
periods of stay and administration of lower overall doses of medication (1). A problem arises, of course, if sufficient staff are not available to be observing the patient on an hourly basis for the moderate
withdrawal not requiring intensive care treatment. Thus, fixed dosing may be required even in an inpatient population. It is a dilemma
that many hospitals face. For inpatient dosing regimens, the general rule is to administer the amount of medication necessary to
suppress autonomic symptoms. Doses in excess of 3 mg/h i.v. initially in individuals in the throes of DTs are not uncommon. Such
patients require close medical monitoring and medication management based strictly on individual patient needs. An example of a
typical outpatient detoxification regimen is given in Table 5-3.

Let us say Bill T. and his wife returned the next day.

CASE 5-2A

*In one scenario, he is shaky, but has managed to go without any
alcohol. Again, his blood pressure is elevated at 142/105, heart
rate 110, temperature is 99.6°F. He has had no vomiting and his
wife was able to get him to eat something. The lorazepam is kept
at the same dose for the next 24 hours. The next day, Bill T. indicates he slept through the night. Although he does not feel well, he
feels better than the day before. The weaning protocol is resumed.*

In the other scenario, Bill T. and his wife return.

CASE 5-2B

*Bill states he drank the night before. Ordinarily he drinks a fifth
of whiskey and a six-pack of beer. He states, and his wife con-
curs, that he drank no more than four beers in the entire preceding 24 hours. He states he found the lorazepam wore off after
about 3 hours, and a beer was enough to hold him over until the
next dose of lorazepam. His vital signs are within normal range
and his breathalyzer is zero.*

Now the clinician faces a dilemma. The decision regarding how
to proceed will depend on the clinician, level of comfort and experience in dealing with such situations, and the alternatives available. Some clinicians, based on the patient's having continued to
drink, would refuse to attempt further outpatient detoxification.

Table 5-3.   Examples of alcohol detoxification regimens[a]

Schedule	Medication[b]

Day 1:
Breathalyzer
Check HR/BP/temperature
  Elevated? Test dose of
    lorazepam (1 mg)
Recheck vital signs in 30 min
  Normal or significant response?
    Give prescription for 24 h
  No or insignificant response?
    Repeat test dose
  No response? Consider
    hospitalization
	Lorazepam 1 mg q4–6 h,
	  depending on degree of
	  tremors, hypertension,
	  tachycardia
	Thiamine 100 mg
	Folic acid 1 mg
	Multivitamin

Day 2: Monitor HR/BP/temperature Based on first day's needs	Lorazepam 1 mg q6 h Thiamine 100 mg Folic acid 1 mg Multivitamin
Day 3: Monitor HR/BP/temperature	Lorazepam 1 mg q8 h Thiamine 100 mg Folic acid 1 mg
Day 4: Monitor HR/BP/temperature	Lorazepam 1 mg q12 h Thiamine 100 mg Folic acid 1 mg Multivitamin

Day 5–7:
(If vital signs have normalized,
  as they usually will have
  done by this point)
	Lorazepam 1 mg qhs
	Thiamine 100 mg
	Folic acid 1 mg
	Multivitamin

HR, heart rate; BP, blood pressure.
[a]The above schedule is only one of a number of possible medication schedules that could be followed. Dosing must be modified daily, based on the patient's response to the previous day's medications, appearance, and concerns. In addition, the clinician would need to be prepared to refer the patient to an inpatient location should any problems arise.
[b]Only 1-day's worth of medication should be given at a time and patient should be required to return daily for monitoring.

Others would attempt to continue, but stop if the patient does not stop drinking immediately. If a detoxification center or other similar facility is available, referral would be a reasonable option. Finally, an inpatient stay for detoxification might be a reasonable suggestion, although difficult to access, given the patient's lack of resources. Table 5-3 shows outpatient detoxification regimens.

MARIJUANA

Withdrawal from cannabis, although not life-threatening, is nevertheless uncomfortable. Withdrawal is characterized by ag-

Table 5-4. Signs and symptoms of early marijuana abstinence (withdrawal)

Tremor
Sweating
Vomiting
Irritability
Sleep disturbance
Nystagmus
Nausea
Diarrhea
Anorexia

itation, restlessness, sleep disturbance, nausea, and intense craving for the drug (7). Whereas the most intense effects are usually over within 7 days, many users describe intense longing for the drug for a much more protracted time period, possibly caused by a slow decrease in levels over an extended period of time. In addition, the sleep disturbance will continue for an extended period of time.

Treatment with medication during this time period is controversial. Some believe it should not be treated at all. The rationale for refusing to treat the early period of cannabis abstinence is that, physiologically, it is time-limited and does not pose any particular threat to the individual. In addition, concern is that jumping to action may send the message that everything that happens has to be treated with a drug—not the message one wants to send. Some believe in giving some symptomatic relief of the discomfort attendant on this period, pointing out that the individual will feel better, function more adequately, may be more likely to engage, and possibly increase the ability to maintain abstinence, although data are lacking to support this latter contention.

If medication is given for the irritability and sleep disturbance, low dose trazodone (25 mg) twice daily and (50–100 mg) at bedtime would be a reasonable choice. Table 5-4 lists the signs and symptoms of early marijuana abstinence.

COCAINE

Typical crack cocaine users use the drug repeatedly during one time interval (a "run"), stopping when the money to buy more drug or the drug itself runs out, at which point they will "crash." The crash after a cocaine run is characterized by exhaustion with fitful sleep, depression, and increased appetite.

Paranoia and violent behavior can occur in the context of cocaine intoxication. They can continue, however, into the period immediately after stopping cocaine use. Sleep disturbance and affective lability are much more prominent symptoms of this period, however. The individual withdrawing from cocaine may be found to sleep constantly, although this is not a restful sleep. Instead, the individual wakes often, is restless, and may be irritable as

Table 5-5.   Signs and symptoms of cocaine withdrawal

Irritability
Prolonged, restless sleep
Increased appetite
+/– Psychosis
Intense fatigue
Depression
+/– Suicidal ideation

well. A profound and even life-threatening depression may set in. It is imperative to assess the individual's risk of self-harm during this time. Hospitalization may be necessary if suicidal ideation is strong enough. The risk of suicide cannot be overstated (8). The period of depression, if it is solely caused by cocaine use, is time-limited, usually lasting less than 3 days.

A wide variety of withdrawal schemes have been tried for the early cocaine withdrawal period, none of which is supported by good data. Bromocriptine and amantadine, for their dopamine-increasing capacity, and desipramine (9–14) for its ability to increase noradrenergic function, have all been given to counter the effects of cocaine withdrawal and, possibly, to decrease craving for the drug. All have found some limited support in the literature, but the side effects of bromocriptine and amantadine, and the need for gradual upward titration of desipramine, are reasons none has gained widespread acceptance. In addition, meta-analysis fails to support the use of antidepressants and dopaminergic agents alike.

Despite the lack of good evidence of efficacy, many clinicians still do use medication to counter some of the irritability and restlessness characteristic of this time. Low dose trazodone (25 mg) three times daily and (50–100 mg) at bedtime has been used for this purpose, as has diphenhydramine, again at doses of 25 mg three times daily and 50 mg at bedtime. The argument for this is, possibly, to help retain the patient in treatment and, thereby, increase the chance of obtaining and maintaining abstinence. Table 5-5 lists the signs and symptoms of cocaine withdrawal.

HEROIN

The appearance of opioid withdrawal has been well recognized for centuries. Withdrawal from all opioids is similar, with onset and conclusion dependent on the half-life of the specific agent. Heroin is the prototype discussed here.

Because of its relatively short half-life, withdrawal from heroin will start after 6 hours of cessation of use in the opioid-dependent individual. Withdrawal typically begins with sweating and generalized discomfort, accompanied by rhinorrhea, lacrimation, and yawning. This is followed by piloerection, aching (especially in the back and joints), muscle twitching, nausea, vomiting, and diarrhea. It is from the presence of the piloerection (gooseflesh) that

Table 5-6.   Signs and symptoms of opiate withdrawal

Pupillary dilation
Increased heart rate
Lacrimation
Nausea
Diarrhea
Sleep disturbance
Initial increase in blood pressure
Piloerection
Rhinorrhea
Vomiting
Yawning
Muscle spasms

the term "cold turkey" is used to describe the opioid withdrawal syndrome. Likewise, the explosive muscle spasms are the source of the term "kicking the habit." Symptoms peak by about 72 hours and have generally subsided by 5 days. Onset is delayed for 2 to 3 days in methadone withdrawal and prolonged for up to a couple of weeks.

Insomnia is a problem both during and in the period after withdrawal. The duration of this symptom is variable and can be long. It is common for individuals who are dependent on opioids as well as a number of other drugs, to complain of significant sleep disturbance.

In an otherwise healthy individual, opioid withdrawal is not a life-threatening entity, although clearly a miserable experience. Problems that arise are typically related to hypovolemia and to electrolyte imbalances that occur as a result. The signs and symptoms of opiate withdrawal are shown in Table 5-6.

WITHDRAWAL REGIMENS

A variety of withdrawal schemes have been developed over the years, all with greater or lesser efficacy. Arguably, the simplest withdrawal scheme is to replace a short-acting opioid (e.g., heroin) with a longer acting opioid (e.g., methadone) and to taper this one. Very stringent laws regarding methadone, however, limit the ability for many facilities to use this approach. Virtually any opioid can be given to counter the symptoms of opioid withdrawal, including morphine, codeine, propoxyphene and hydrocodone should a compelling medical reason exist for doing so. It should be noted, however, that it is illegal to use a narcotic other than methadone for opioid maintenance or withdrawal and then only in the context of a federally licensed methadone program. This means that if a heroin addict is placed on codeine, for example, to keep that person out of withdrawal, the law has been broken. For an exhaustive review of methadone issues and answers, see the following: the Federal Regulation of Methadone Treatment: Executive Summary by Richard Rettig and Adam Yarmolinsky, National Academy Press, 1995; or *www.methadone.org/fedregs.html*.

Recognizing that not every facility has a methadone license, but may have need to attempt detoxification of the opioid-dependent addict, a popular approach to opioid detoxification is discussed below. It should be noted, however, that in individuals using high doses of heroin daily, this approach is unlikely to provide significant symptom relief. Potency and costs vary from place to place, but a general rule is that among individuals with a habit costing in excess of $50/day, the patient is likely to have a difficult course if the following is the only medication offered. The patient is likely to suffer significant distress and have a great deal of fluid loss requiring fluid replacement or hospitalization as a result. In addition, it should be noted that clonidine abuse among opioid-dependent individuals has been described in the literature and may be more common than has been thought (15–17).

Tramadol, a synthetic μ-agonist has also proved to be of significant benefit in withdrawing individuals from opioid use. This medication itself can cause tolerance and withdrawal and, therefore, should be given with caution, and dispensed only in small quantities. Patients should receive 25 to 50 mg every 6 hours for up to 48 hours, and the dose gradually decreased over 4 to 6 days. Extreme caution is advised if the patient is on a serotonin reuptake inhibiting antidepressant, as fatalities have occurred when such a combination has been used.

Pregnancy

It is not recommended that opioid-dependent pregnant women be permitted to go into withdrawal. Rather, the predominant recommendation is that they be placed on methadone for the duration of the pregnancy, as noted in Chapter 4. Clonidine is also theoretically contraindicated in pregnancy because of the possibility of decreasing placental perfusion and depriving the fetus of oxygen. Stress is placed on the term "theoretically," as a review of the literature failed to turn up any reports of problems associated with intentional or inadvertent clonidine administration to a pregnant opioid-addicted woman. In the event that for some reason withdrawal is necessary, the safest time for both mother and fetus is during the mid trimester.

Opioid Withdrawal Regimen

One particular opioid withdrawal regimen has been popular for two decades. It combines the use of clonidine, either orally or transdermally; dicyclomine for abdominal discomfort; an antiemetic, if the need should arise; an antidiarrheal agent, if necessary; and a nonsteroidal antiinflammatory analgesic on a routine basis for the aching that inevitably occurs. This particular regimen has been published widely and used extensively and will not be repeated here. For individuals with a mild to moderate pattern of opioid usage, this regimen has some merit in reducing the severity of symptoms. For addicted patients using large quantities of opioids or needing to use, for example, heroin more than twice a day, the discomfort the patient feels will be severe and this detoxification regimen is unlikely to be of much benefit. Such a patient would do much better with tramadol or referral to a methadone clinic for a methadone withdrawal. Table 5-7 summarizes some of the discussion above.

Table 5-7. Substance withdrawal

Substance	Onset	Duration	Heart Rate	Blood Pressure	Body Temperature	Other Signs and Symptoms	Detoxification Strategy[a]
Alcohol	12–36 hr decrease in alcohol level	3–7 days	Increased	Increased	Slight increase	Nausea, vomiting, diarrhea, headache, seizures, hallucinations, sleep disturbance	Lorazepam, 1 mg every 6 hr on a decreasing basis Thiamine 100 mg every day[b] Folic acid, 1 mg every day Multivitamin with iron every day
Heroin	4–6 hr	3–6 days	Increased	Initial increase, then decrease caused by hypovolemia		Nausea, vomiting, diarrhea, lacrimation, rhinorrhea, piloerection, muscle spasms, sleep disturbance	Tramadol, clonidine regimen Methadone
Cocaine		3 days	Slight decrease	Slight decrease	Slight decrease	Irritability, sleep disturbance, paranoia, depression, risk of suicide	Trazodone 25 as needed and 50–100 qhs

[a]Do not begin detoxification in a pregnant female.
[b]Thiamine must be given before giving glucose.

REFERENCES
1. Saitz R, Friedman L, Mayo-Smith M. Alcohol withdrawal: a nationwide survey of inpatient treatment practices. *J Gen Intern Med* 1995;10(9):479–487.
2. Mayo-Smith MF. Pharmacological management of alcohol withdrawal: a meta analysis and evidence-based practice guideline. *JAMA* 1997;278(2):144–151.
3. Schuckit MA. Alcohol and alcoholism. In: Braunwald E, Fauci AS, Kasper DL, et al. *Harrison's principles of internal medicine,* 15th ed. New York: McGraw-Hill, 2001: 2561–2566.
4. Maier SE, Chen WJ, Miller JA, et al. Fetal alcohol exposure and temporal vulnerability regional differences in alcohol induced microencephaly as a function of the timing of binge like exposure during rat brain development. *Alcohol Clin Exp Res* 1997;21(8): 1418–1428.
5. Seidl JJ, Layde P. Lorazepam to prevent alcohol withdrawal seizures. *J Fam Pract* 1999;48(8):575–576.
6. Chance J. Emergency department treatment of alcohol withdrawal seizures with phenytoin. *Ann Emerg Med* 1991;20(5):520–522.
7. Mendelson JH, Mello NK. Cocaine and other commonly abused drugs. In: Braunwald E, Fauci AS, Kasper DL, et al. *Harrison's principles of internal medicine,* 15th ed. New York: McGraw-Hill, 2001:2571–2574.
8. Marzuk PM, Tardiff K, Leon AC, et al. Prevalence of cocaine use among residents of New York City who committed suicide during a one-year period. *Am J Psychiatry* 1992;149(3):371–375.
9. Kosten TR, Morgan CM, Flacione J, et al. Pharmacotherapy for cocaine abusing methadone maintained patients using amantadine or desipramine. *Arch Gen Psychiatry* 1992;49(11):894–898.
10. Tennant FS, Rawson RA. Cocaine and amphetamine dependence treated with desipramine. *NIDA Res Monogr* 1983;43:351–355.
11. Campbell JL, Thomas HM, Gabrielli W, et al. Impact of desipramine or carbamazepine on patient retention in outpatient cocaine treatment: preliminary findings. *J Addict Dis* 1994;13(4): 191–199.
12. Hall SM, Tunis S, Triffleman E, et al. Continuity of care and desipramine in primary cocaine abusers. *J Nerv Ment Dis* 1994;182 (10):570–575.
13. Weddington WW, Brown BS, Haertzen CA, et al. Comparison of amantadine and desipramine combined with psychotherapy for treatment of cocaine dependence. *Am J Drug Alcohol Abuse* 1991; 17(2):1137–1152.
14. Tennant FS, Sagherian AA. Double blind comparison of amantadine and bromocriptine for ambulatory withdrawal from cocaine dependence. *Arch Intern Med* 1987;147:109–112.
15. Dennison SJ. Abuse of clonidine by opiate addicts. *Psychiatr Q* 2001;72(2):191–195.
16. Agelink MD, Dammers S, Zeit T. Clonidine—a risk of abuse in psychiatric patients? *Nervenarzt* 1996;67(3):253–255.
17. Beuger M, Tommasello A, Schwartz R, et al. Clonidine use and abuse among methadone program applicants and patients. *J Subst Abuse Treat* 1998;15(6):589–593.

Schizophrenia and Substance Misuse

1. Background
   a. Of the population, 1% with problem
   b. Demographics
      i. Men more than women
      ii. Onset late teens, early twenties
   c. Increased risk of suicide
2. Medication issues
   a. Noncompliance great
   b. Discontinuation increases relapse
   c. Typical antipsychotics affect positive symptoms more than negative
   d. Atypical antipsychotics have better affect on positive symptoms
3. Substance use and schizophrenia
   a. Dual diagnosis common in schizophrenia
   b. Consequences of substance use
      i. Increased rate of hospitalization
      ii. Earlier age of onset of psychosis
      iii. Alcohol worsens overall prognosis
      iv. Detection of substance use disorder difficult
4. Schizophrenia and nicotine
   a. Very high incidence of nicotine use
   b. Nicotine improves negative symptoms of disorder
   c. Nicotine induces metabolism of typical antipsychotics (i.e., reduces efficacy)
5. Schizophrenia and alcohol
   a. Good data difficult because often combined with information on marijuana use
   b. Worsens prognosis of schizophrenia
   c. Much higher suicide rate
6. Schizophrenia and marijuana
   a. Good data difficult because often combined with information on alcohol use
   b. Effect of marijuana variable and can be dose related
   c. Can induce psychosis at higher doses: problem of what constitutes "high" dose
7. Schizophrenia and cocaine
   a. Very high rate of cocaine use; much higher than among healthy population and apparently rising in frequency
   b. Not clear that cocaine use definitely worsens long-term outcome of condition
   c. Cocaine use worsens positive symptoms, induces psychosis, but improves negative symptoms
8. Antipsychotics and drugs of abuse
   a. Nicotine
      i. Induces metabolism of typical antipsychotics
      ii. Abrupt discontinuation of nicotine can result in akathisia
      iii. Clozapine plus nicotine patch may decrease smoking
   b. Alcohol
      i. No known cases of fatalities caused by the combination of antipsychotics and alcohol alone
      ii. High-potency antipsychotics and alcohol reasonably safe combination
      iii. Low-potency neuroleptics and alcohol only theoretic risk
   c. Cocaine
      i. In combination with high-potency neuroleptics, can increase risk of neuroleptic malignant syndrome and dystonias

ii.   Clozapine decreases appetite for cocaine but must be used with caution because of potential for risk of seizure and syncope

d.   Opioids

i.   Opioid use in this population uncommon

ii.   Opioids may improve negative symptoms of schizophrenia

iii.   Some risk of competitive inhibition between antipsychotics and opioid preparations, thus a balance must be struck.

BACKGROUND

Approximately 1% of the population of the United States has schizophrenia. The ravages of the disease are felt throughout the lifetime of the patient, as the symptoms of schizophrenia appear in the late teens and early twenties. Men, who are diagnosed with the disorder significantly more often than women, may have an onset of the disease at a younger age, although some dispute this (1,2).

As with substance dependence, schizophrenia is a chronic, relapsing, and progressive disease. Three quarters of those with schizophrenia will have recurrent psychotic episodes: most have their first relapse to psychosis within 2 years of initial presentation (3–5). The same percentage of patients, however, will show improvement in these symptoms when treated with antipsychotic medication (6).

Individuals with schizophrenia have a suicide rate nine times that of an age-matched control group. Death by other violent means is also higher than for the general population. Comorbid substance use pushes both rates even higher irrespective of gender (7–11).

ETIOLOGY

Clearly, a hereditary component to schizophrenia exists. Schizophrenia occurs in first-degree relatives of schizophrenic patients at a rate ten times that of the normal population. Environmental factors can also contribute to the occurrence of schizophrenia. The disorder occurs in individuals born in winter slightly more often than people born at other times. An increased rate of schizophrenia has also been found to occur in children born to women during times of famine (12–14).

It is not possible to predict with any certainty who will develop schizophrenia. Both retrospective and prospective studies, however, have identified premorbid characteristics of individuals who go on to develop the full syndrome of schizophrenia. Traits such as poor sociability, delayed fine and gross motor skills, and speech and educational difficulties have all been identified as early signs of schizophrenia and suggestive of neurologic involvement (15–18).

An obvious question is whether early intervention, even before the onset of symptoms, might prevent the disease entirely or improve outcome from this debilitating disorder. The problem, however, is that antipsychotics are powerful medications that affect multiple organ and neurotransmitter systems. The older ones had numerous side effects and the consequences of long-term use of the newer ones are unknown. An ethical dilemma yet to be resolved is whether it is justifiable to expose young people to such risks when they only theoretically might develop the disease (19,20).

MEDICATION RESPONSE

Treatment of any medical or psychiatric disorder is compromised by noncompliance with prescribed medication, and such is definitely the case with schizophrenia. Slightly more than half of individuals with schizophrenia who are prescribed antipsychotic medications actually take them and far fewer take them as prescribed (21). Unlike some other conditions, however, discontinuing medication for schizophrenia increases the rate of relapse by at least fivefold. Making the issue of medication noncompliance even more pressing is that the longer and more frequently the individual is psychotic, the lower the overall response may be to medication (6).

Historically, the symptoms of schizophrenia have been broken down into "positive" and "negative" types. The so-called "typical" antipsychotics are well known to affect the positive symptoms much more than the negative. Both the percentage of responders and the degree of relief of negative symptoms may improve with the advent of atypical antipsychotics, which have a different efficacy profile than do the more typical medications. With typical antipsychotics, the greatest degree of symptomatic improvement occurs in the first 6 weeks to 6 months of treatment (6). With the atypical antipsychotics, on the other hand, improvement can continue well past this point (6). Interestingly, a gender difference exists in regard to medication response. Evidence suggests that women may respond more completely to antipsychotics than do men and at lower overall average doses of medication (2) (Table 6-1).

SUBSTANCE MISUSE AND SCHIZOPHRENIA

Misuse of psychoactive substances is the norm, not the exception, among individuals with schizophrenia, according to studies in the United States, Canada, and Europe. In addition, the use of illicit substances, especially cocaine, may be increasing among this group, although it has plateaued in the remainder of the population (22). Estimates are that from one quarter to as many of two thirds of individuals with schizophrenia have a comorbid substance use disorder. In fact, schizophrenia ranks second among all psychiatric conditions as being associated with substance use disorders. Even when socioeconomic factors (e.g., poverty,

Table 6-1. Gender differences in schizophrenia

	Males	Females
Age at onset or diagnosis	Earlier	Later
Percentage	60–70	30–40
Course of illness	No gender difference	No gender difference
Average medication dosage	Higher	Lower
Response to medication	Less complete than females	More complete than males

unemployment, little education) are taken into consideration, dual diagnosis remains disproportionately high among individuals with schizophrenia (23–26).

Psychosis can present at a slightly earlier age among individuals with schizophrenia and comorbid substance use disorders than among those with only schizophrenia (27). The dually diagnosed tend to be hospitalized more often as well. Interestingly, no clear evidence shows that the severity of schizophrenic symptoms or long-term functioning is substantially worsened by the presence of substance misuse, with the notable exception of alcohol, which worsens the prognosis overall (28,29).

Detecting the presence of a substance use disorder in the face of schizophrenia can be difficult. Instruments commonly used to make the diagnosis of substance abuse or dependence (e.g., "CAGE" [cut down, annoyed by criticism, guilty about drinking, eye-opener drinks] questionnaire, the "mini-MAST [Michigan Alcoholism Screening Test]," and the "Addiction Severity Index"), may not be reliable in this population. One group found that the more sick the individual being interviewed was, the less likely that person was to disclose the information asked by these instruments (30,31).

Schizophrenia, by itself, increases the likelihood of an individual being homeless or incarcerated. Having this illness, regardless of gender, increases the likelihood the individual will come into contact with the legal system for a variety of infractions, including an increased risk of violence, most of which occurs after the onset of the mental illness. When the individual concomitantly suffers from a substance use disorder, however, the risk of violence is drastically increased (32–35). It should be borne in mind, however, that despite the increased risk of violence, the actual percentage of violent crimes committed by this population is actually low. Further, control of psychotic symptoms results in a decrease in violent activity (36–38).

Finally, the rate of suicide, already increased among individuals with schizophrenia, is further increased by comorbidity (7,11,39–41) (Table 6-2).

SCHIZOPHRENIA AND NICOTINE

People who abuse alcohol or any other drug are likely to abuse nicotine, and people who use nicotine are likely to use alcohol and other drugs. These facts hold true regardless of the population examined. Among individuals with schizophrenia, the prevalence of nicotine abuse is markedly high. In the United States, approximately one third of the general population smokes tobacco (42,43). Globally, more than 50% up to 90% of persons with schizophrenia smoke tobacco, and those who smoke tend to smoke heavily (43–47).

A variety of theories have been offered to explain this phenomenon. The simplest is that, given the ravages the disease and its impact on the quality of life, smoking may be one of the only sources of pleasure the individual with schizophrenia has. Such reasoning may explain why little effort has been made to curb smoking among the chronically mentally ill until the last decade (44,48–50).

The finding that nicotine speeds the rate of metabolism of antipsychotic drugs has given rise to a different theory. Perhaps the individual is unwittingly (or intentionally) lowering drug levels of antipsychotics, thereby reducing uncomfortable side effects. In

6. Schizophrenia and Substance Misuse 73

**Table 6-2. Comparison: Not dually diagnosed
vs. dually diagnosed schizophrenia**

	Schizophrenia Alone	Dually Diagnosed Schizophrenia
Age at diagnosis	Slightly older	Slightly younger
Risk of criminal activity	Greater than general population	Much greater than general population
Risk of violence	Greater than general population	Much greater than general population
Rate of hospitalization	Lower	Higher
Length of hospitalization	No difference[a]	No difference[a]
Long-term outcome	No difference[a]	No difference[a]

[a]With exception of alcohol

fact, some evidence suggests that typical antipsychotics actually increase the rate of tobacco use in some individuals with schizophrenia (51). This argument is weakened by the fact that individuals with a first episode of psychosis and no prior exposure to medications smoke at the same rate as those with a long history of schizophrenia (45–47).

New research offers a very different view. Although individuals with schizophrenia who also use nicotine require much higher than average doses of neuroleptic medication for symptom control, when compared with nonsmokers with the disorder, they also demonstrate fewer cognitive effects when they receive haloperidol. In addition, nicotine use significantly reduces the negative symptoms of schizophrenia, suggesting two very positive therapeutic effects (52–54).

SCHIZOPHRENIA AND ALCOHOL

Data regarding the effect of alcohol alone on schizophrenia are difficult to come by, as most studies group marijuana and alcohol together. Many studies from the United States and Europe have found that marijuana and alcohol are the substances most abused next to tobacco by schizophrenics, but fail to differentiate the effects of each. From 25% to 50% of individuals with schizophrenia have comorbid alcohol use disorders, the presence of which is associated with greatly increased positive symptoms (29,55–57).

With many substances, little evidence indicates that the long-term course of schizophrenia is worsened by their abuse. Alcohol, however, is different. Persons with schizophrenia and alcohol dependence have a poorer prognosis overall than do those who do not abuse or use other drugs. They tend toward more and longer hospitalizations, poorer out-of-hospital functioning, and have a higher suicide rate than users of other substances (58–60). Possibly, many of the differences simply result from the physical and cognitive changes that alcohol causes in general, as opposed to a unique influence of this drug on schizophrenia. As noted in Chapter 4, next to nicotine, alcohol is the drug of abuse with the most toxic effects on the body.

SCHIZOPHRENIA AND MARIJUANA

As noted, individuals with schizophrenia who abuse alcohol tend to abuse marijuana and vice versa. In general, where marijuana abuse is examined, it is ordinarily in combination with alcohol, with no effort to differentiate the effects of each. Although the number of studies is not extensive, some trends can be discerned in regard to the effect of marijuana on the course of this illness.

Frequency of marijuana use ties, or is slightly ahead of, the frequency with which alcohol is abused by individuals with schizophrenia, according to studies both in Europe and in North America. As with alcohol, marijuana use is associated with an increased frequency of relapse to psychosis. Further, this effect is dose dependent. Low doses of tetrahydrocannabinol, defined as less than or one marijuana cigarette per day, may not cause significant problems among those with schizophrenia. It is clear, however, that among those with schizophrenia as well as in normal individuals with no history of premorbid psychosis, a high overall daily dosage of δ-9 tetrahydrocannabinol (THC) increases the likelihood of psychotic symptoms and of rehospitalization (61).

CASE 6-1

Chris C., 20, had his first hospitalization at the age of 19 years. At admission, his urine was positive for marijuana, and the smell of alcohol was on his breath. Given a diagnosis of "substance-induced psychosis," he was given no medications during his hospital stay, and his condition gradually cleared sufficiently to be discharged back to his family. He was back less than a month later. His family indicated he "hadn't been right" since being discharged. Once home, they reported he spent most of his time in his room in the dark. He could be heard talking, sometimes quite loudly, although they knew no one was with him. In addition, he didn't wash, had to be cajoled into eating, and seemed to distrust everyone around him.

This time, his urine drug screen was negative and his family indicated he rarely went out, making it unlikely that he was drinking to any significant degree. With his continued odd behavior and apparent auditory hallucinations in the absence of current substance abuse, he was given a diagnosis of schizophrenia and medication was begun.

Over the years, Chris C., now 24, responded well to several medications, both typical and atypical. His compliance with any medication regimen, however, was poor. His usual pattern was to leave the hospital, discontinue his medication and return to using street drugs and alcohol. Because of his ongoing substance use, some physicians were reluctant to put him on a depot neuroleptic, fearing that a drug interaction might occur.

SCHIZOPHRENIA AND OPIATES

The most impressive finding regarding the effect of opiate abuse on schizophrenia is that, in general, individuals with schizophrenia do not use opiates. Although European studies differ in regard to the exact percentage of persons with schizophrenia and comorbid opiate dependency problems, in the United States it appears that opiate abuse among those with schizophrenia is low, and much lower than among the general population. Reports are found of methadone-maintained individuals becoming psychotic during withdrawal from this medication and then show improvement in symptoms when the opiate is reinstated. This suggests that opiates themselves have antipsychotic properties, but does not explain why persons with schizophrenia would avoid it (62). Some researchers suggest that maintaining a heroin habit requires a higher level of functioning than many persons with schizophrenia are capable of achieving. For example, as noted in Chapter 4, heroin, with its brief half-life, requires two to four times per day use just to stay out of withdrawal once the user is physiologically dependent. Perhaps persons with schizophrenia in general are not able to develop sufficient organized behavior to obtain the drug reliably. Veterans' Hospital methadone programs appear to have more maintenance patients with schizophrenia than other programs. This may well represent a unique and select population that is uncharacteristic of individuals with schizophrenia in general. Regardless of the reason, opioid dependence among this population is an uncommon finding (63–65).

SCHIZOPHRENIA AND PSYCHOSTIMULANTS

On the opposite end of the spectrum from schizophrenia and opiates, psychostimulant abuse is several times higher in this population than in the general population. In fact, the rate of cocaine use, in particular, may be increasing among persons with schizophrenia at the same time that it appears to be at a plateau or decreasing among other groups. In addition, several studies suggested that the use of cocaine by schizophrenics increases according to length of exposure to, and dosage of, neuroleptic medications (22,66).

Frequency of psychotic episodes and numbers of hospitalizations are undeniably increased among persons with schizophrenia who use cocaine. In addition, persons with cocaine habits require higher average doses of antipsychotic medication following recent cocaine use than do nonusers. This is not, however, a permanent condition. Following periods of abstinence, medication requirements fall and are similar to those of nonusers. In addition, symptom severity and long-term outcome have not been found to be significantly different between persons with schizophrenia who do or do not use cocaine (67–69).

It appears that not all of the effects of cocaine on schizophrenia are negative. At the same time that this drug increases the positive symptoms resulting in a worsening of psychosis, just as with nicotine, cocaine use is associated with significant improvement in negative symptoms. Thus, those who claim an increase in sociability and an ability to relate better to the environment, in fact, are correctly reporting the effect the drug has on their functioning (70,71) (Table 6-3).

Table 6-3. Substance *vs.* schizophrenia

	Age at Onset of sxs	Frequency of Hospitalization	Severity of Negative sxs	Severity of Positive sys	Medication Effect	Long-term Outcome
Nicotine			Improves negative sxs		Increases drug needs (↑metabolism)	No difference
Alcohol	Alcohol use follows sxs onset	Increases hospitalization rate			Potential for interaction greater with less potent typical antipsychotics No fatalities in literature	Generally worse prognosis
Marijuana	Use follows onset	Low dose marijuana no change Medium or high dose increases hospitalization		Low dose no change Medium or high dose worsens sys		

	Cocaine use follows sxs onset	Increases frequency of hospitalization	Improves negative sxs	Worsens positive sxs	↑Risk of NMS and dystonic reactions with high potency typical antipsychotics	No change
Cocaine	No data	Increases frequency of hospitalization	Improves negative sxs	Worsens positive sxs	↑Risk of NMS and dystonic reactions with high potency typical antipsychotics	No change
Opiates	No data	No data	No data	No data	Methadone can augment antipsychotics, improve symptoms	No data

NMS, neuroleptic malignant syndrome; sxs, signs; sys, symptoms.

MEDICATION EFFECTS

Although individuals with schizophrenia receive a variety of different psychotropic medications, the principal medications under discussion here are the antipsychotics, typical and atypical, and how they interact with substances of abuse. Discussion of antidepressants and mood stabilizers are found in chapters on depression and bipolar illness, respectively.

Nicotine

As noted, nicotine increases the metabolism of typical antipsychotics, thereby reducing their effectiveness. This can present a real problem for patients when they are hospitalized in facilities where smoking is not permitted. They may suffer an abrupt increase in neuroleptic level because of the absence of competitive inhibition (72). Clinicians, then, should be aware that these patients can become over medicated on the same doses of medication that were previously therapeutic and uncomfortable as a result because of akathisia and other extrapyramidal reactions. In addition, these same medications can actually be related to an increase in smoking among individuals with schizophrenia (51). Clozapine, alone or in combination with nicotine patches, has been shown to result in a modest reduction in tobacco use (38,48,73). However, McCarthy (74) reported the case of a patient on clozapine who suffered a seizure when he was forced to abruptly cease his nicotine use. This was attributed to a sudden rise in his clozapine level caused by the absence of nicotine (74).

Alcohol

Traditionally, the use of alcohol by persons on major tranquilizers has been a source of tremendous concern because of the possible interaction of the two. Although this is not a concern to be dismissed lightly, the comprehensive review of drug interactions by Barnhill (74a) does not list case reports of interactions between alcohol and antipsychotic medications, although they do cite experimental evidence noting significant additive effects with typical antipsychotics. This concern has been one reason that clinicians have withheld medication from patients who were actively drinking. To date, no cases are reported of a lethal interaction of a high-potency neuroleptic in combination with alcohol alone. The problem comes in regard to multiple medications. Always keep in mind that individuals on antipsychotics often receive multiple medications, and that some of those drugs may prove lethal in combination with alcohol. An example is the case report of the death of an individual using alcohol who was also receiving haloperidol and diazepam (75).

Psychostimulants

Cocaine use presents considerable problems for the treating clinician in terms of antipsychotic selection. A number of case reports have been filed that seem to show that this drug significantly increases the risk of dystonic reactions, especially when given in conjunction with haloperidol (76–81). A further concern has been raised that this combination also poses an increased risk for neuroleptic malignant syndrome (82).

In keeping with the finding that clozapine appears to decrease substance use among individuals with schizophrenia,

Farren et al. (83) administered this medication to patients to assess the safety of clozapine in combination with cocaine. Patients reported a decrease in the subjective experience to cocaine, generally without a dramatic change in vital signs. However, they also demonstrated an increase in serum cocaine levels. The researchers further noted that one patient also experienced a near syncopal reaction when clozapine was administered in the presence of cocaine.

Another study showed that the atypical antipsychotic, risperidone, decreased craving for cocaine among drug users who were not schizophrenic. Whereas it does appear to have some efficacy in this population, the dropout rate among subjects in the study was exorbitant, making this approach seem impractical. In addition, its applicability to the dually diagnosed with schizophrenia is unknown (84,85).

Opioids

As noted, opiate dependence in a population with schizophrenia is unusual. The combination of opiates with antipsychotics is not, however, and has been exploited for enhancing analgesia. In addition, as noted, opiates have been shown to have antipsychotic properties in their own right. As an augmentation strategy in individuals with schizophrenia who are poorly responsive to neuroleptic medication, methadone, for example, has been found to result in significant symptomatic improvement (86). Conversely, case reports have shown risperidone precipitating withdrawal symptoms in individuals on stable maintenance doses of methadone (87).

For a review of substances of abuse and interactions with antipsychotic medications, see Chapter 16.

REFERENCES

1. Kendler KS, Walsh D. Gender and schizophrenia: results of an epidemiologically based family study. *Br J Psychiatry* 1995;167(2): 184–192.
2. Szymanski S, Lieberman JA, Alvir JM, et al. Gender differences in onset of illness treatment response, course and biologic indexes in first episode schizophrenic patients. *Am J Psychiatry* 1995; 152(5):698–703.
3. Breier A, Schreiber JL, Dyer J, et al. National Institute of Mental Health longitudinal study of chronic schizophrenia. *Arch Gen Psychiatry* 1991;48:239–246.
4. Eaton WW, Bilker W, Haro JM, et al. Long-term course of hospitalization for schizophrenia. Part II: Change with passage of time. *Schizophr Bull* 1992;18(2):229–241.
5. Eaton WW, Mortensen PB, Herrman H, et al. Long-term course of hospitalization for schizophrenia. Part I. Risk for rehospitalization. *Schizophr Bull* 1992;18(2):217–218.
6. Janicak PG. *Handbook of psychopharmacotherapy*. Philadelphia: Lippincott Williams & Wilkins, 1999.
7. Mortensen PB, Juel K. Mortality and causes of death in schizophrenic patients in Denmark. *Acta Psychiatr Scand* 1990;81(4): 372–377.
8. Siris SG. Suicide and schizophrenia. *J Psychopharmacol* 2001; 15(2):127–135.

9. DeHert M, Kwame; M, Peuskens J. Risk factors for suicide in young people suffering from schizophrenia: a long-term follow up study. *Schizophr Res* 2001;47(2):127–134.
10. Rossau CD, Mortensen PB. Risk factors for suicide in patients with schizophrenia: nested case control study. *Br J Psychiatry* 1997;171(10):355–359.
11. Harris EC, Barraclough B. Excess mortality of mental disorder. *Br J Psychiatry* 1998;173(7):11–53.
12. Boyd JH, Pulver AE, Stewart W. Season of birth: schizophrenia and bipolar disorder. *Schizophr Bull* 1986;12(2):173–186.
13. Torrey EF, Miller J, Rawlings R, et al. Seasonality of birth in schizophrenia and bipolar disorder: a review of the literature. *Schizophr Res* 1997;28(1):1–38.
14. Kendell RE, Adams W. Unexplained fluctuations in the risk for schizophrenia by month and year of birth. *Br J Psychiatry* 1991; 158:758–763.
15. Cannon M, Jones P, Gilvarry C, et al. Premorbid social functioning in schizophrenia and bipolar disorder: similarities and differences. *Am J Psychiatry* 1997;154(11):1544–1550.
16. Davidson M, Reichenberg A, Rabinowitz J, et al. Behavioral and intellectual markers for schizophrenia in apparently healthy male adolescents. *Am J Psychiatry* 1999;156(9):1328–1335.
17. Parnas J. From predisposition to psychosis: progression of symptoms in schizophrenia. *Acta Psychiatr Scand Suppl* 1999;99(395): 20–29.
18. Hodges A, Byrne M, Grant E, et al. People at risk of schizophrenia: sample characteristics of the first 100 cases in the Edinburgh High Risk study. *Br J Psychiatry* 1999;174(6):547–553.
19. McGlashan TH. Early detection and intervention of schizophrenia: rationale and research. *Br J Psychiatry* 1998;172(Suppl 33):3–6.
20. Yung AR, Phillips LJ, McGorry PD, et al. Prediction of psychosis: a step towards indicated prevention of schizophrenia. *Br J Psychiatry* 1998;172(Suppl 33):14–20.
21. Cramer JA, Rosenheck R. Enhancing medication compliance for people with serious mental illness. *J Nerv Ment Dis* 1999;187(1): 53–55.
22. LeDuc PA, Mittleman G. Schizophrenia and psychostimulant abuse: a review and re-analysis of clinical evidence. *Psychopharmacology* 1995;121:407–427.
23. Modestin J, Nussbaumer C, Angst K, et al. Use of potentially abusive psychotropic substances in psychiatric inpatients. *Eur Arch Psychiatry Clin Neurosci* 1997;247(3):146–153.
24. Mueser KT, Yarnold PR, Levinson DF, et al. Prevalence of substance abuse in schizophrenia: demographic and clinical correlates. *Schizophr Bull* 1990;16(1):31–54.
25. Chouljian JL, Shumway M, Balancio E, et al. Substance use among schizophrenic outpatients: prevalence, course, and relation to functional status. *Ann Clin Psychiatry* 1995;7(1):19–24.
26. Barbee JG, Clark PD, Crapanzana MS, et al. Alcohol and substance abuse among schizophrenic patients presenting to an emergency psychiatry service. *J Nerv Ment Dis* 1989;177(7): 400–406.
27. Addington J, Addington D. Effect of substance misuse in early psychosis. *Br J Psychiatry* 1998;172(Suppl 33):134–136.

28. Brunette MF, Mueser KT, Xie H, et al. Relationships between symptoms of schizophrenia and substance abuse. *J Nerv Ment Dis* 1997;185(1):13–20.
29. Cantwell RB, Glazebrook J, Dalkin C, et al. Prevalence of substance misuse in first episode psychosis. *Br J Psychiatry* 1999; 174(2):150–153.
30. Drake RE, Osher FC, Noordsy DL, et al. Diagnosis of alcohol use disorders in schizophrenia. *Schizophr Bull* 1990;16(1):57–66.
31. Appleby L, Dyson V, Altman E, et al. Assessing substance use in multiproblem patients: reliability and validity of the addiction severity index in a mental hospital population. *J Nerv Ment Dis* 1997;185:159–165.
32. Beaudoin MN, Hodgins S, Lavoie F. Homicide, schizophrenia and substance abuse or dependency. *Can J Psychiatry* 1993;38(8): 541–546.
33. Rasanen P, Tiihonen J, Isohanni M, et al. Schizophrenia, alcohol abuse, and violent behavior: a 26-year follow-up study of an unselected birth cohort. *Schizophr Bull* 1998;24(3):437–441.
34. Coid JW. Dangerous patients with mental illness: increased risks warrant new policies, adequate resources, and appropriate legislation. *BMJ* 1996;312:965–966.
35. Humphreys MS, Johnstone EC, MacMillan JF, et al. Dangerous behavior preceding first admissions for schizophrenia. *Br J Psychiatry* 1992;161:501–505.
36. Steinert T, Sippach T, Gebhardt RP. How common is violence in schizophrenia despite neuroleptic treatment? *Pharmacopsychiatry* 2000;33(3):98–102.
37. Chengappa KN, Levine J, Ulrich R, et al. Impact of risperidone on seclusion and restraint at a state psychiatric hospital. *Can J Psychiatry* 2000;45(9):827–832.
38. Volavka J. The effects of clozapine on aggression and substance abuse in schizophrenic patients. *J Clin Psychiatry* 1999;60(Suppl 12):43–46.
39. Schwartz RC, Cohen BN. Risk factors for suicidality among clients with schizophrenia. *Journal of Counseling and Development* 2001;79(3):314–319.
40. Gut-Fayand A, Dervaux A, Olie J-P, et al. Substance abuse and suicidality in schizophrenia: a common risk factor linked to impulsivity. *Psychiatry Res* 2001;102(1):65–72.
41. DeHert M, McKenzie K, Peuskens J. Risk factors for suicide in young people suffering from schizophrenia: a long-term follow-up study. *Schizophr Res* 2001;47(2–3):127–134.
42. Abuse NIoD. Cigarettes and Other Nicotine Products. Bethesda, MD: National Institute on Drug Abuse, 1999:1–4.
43. deLeon J, Dadvand M, Canuso C, et al. Schizophrenia and smoking: an epidemiological survey in a state hospital. *Am J Psychiatry* 1995;152(3):453–455.
44. Dalack GW, Healy DJ, Meador-Woodruff JH. Nicotine dependence in schizophrenia: clinical phenomena and laboratory findings. *Am J Psychiatry* 1998;155(11):1490–1501.
45. Glassman AH. Cigarette smoking: implications for psychiatric illness. *Am J Psychiatry* 1993;150(4):546–553.
46. Kelly C, McCreadie RG. Smoking habits, current symptoms, and premorbid characteristics of schizophrenic patients in Nithsdale, Scotland. *Am J Psychiatry* 1999;156(11):1751–1757.

47. McEvoy JP, Brown S. Smoking in first episode patients with schizophrenia. *Am J Psychiatry* 1999;156(7):1120–1121.
48. George TP, Ziedonis DM, Feingold A, et al. Nicotine transdermal patch and atypical antipsychotic medications for smoking cessation in schizophrenia. *Am J Psychiatry* 2000;157(11): 1835–1842.
49. Addington J, el-Guebaly N, Campbell W, et al. Smoking cessation treatment for patients with schizophrenia. *Am J Psychiatry* 1998; 155(7):974–976.
50. Itkin O, Nemets B, Einat H. Smoking habits in bipolar and schizophrenic outpatients in southern Israel. *J Clin Psychiatry* 2001; 62(4):269–272.
51. McEvoy JP, Freudenreich O, Levin ED, et al. Haloperidol increases smoking in patients with schizophrenia. *Psychopharmacology* 1995;119(1):124–126.
52. Ernst M, Matochik JA, Heishman SJ, et al. Effect of nicotine on brain activation during performance of a working memory task. *Proc Nat Acad Sci USA* 2001;98(8):4728–4733.
53. Lee C, Frangou S, Russell MA, et al. Effect of haloperidol on nicotine-induced enhancement of vigilance in human subjects. *J Psychopharmacol* 1997;11(3):253–257.
54. Levin ED, Wilson W, Rose JE, et al. Nicotine-haloperidol interactions and cognitive performance in schizophrenics. *Neuropsychopharmacology* 1996;15(5):429–436.
55. Kessler KR, Crum RM, Warner LA, et al. Lifetime co-occurrence of DSM-IIIR alcohol abuse and dependence with other psychiatric disorders in the national comorbidity survey. *Arch Gen Psychiatry* 1997;54(4):313–321.
56. Menezes PR, Johnson S, Thornicroft G, et al. Drug and alcohol problems among individuals with severe mental illness in South London. *Br J Psychiatry* 1996;168:612–619.
57. Regier DA, Farmer ME, Rae DS, et al. Comorbidity of mental disorders with alcohol and other drug abuse: results from the Epidemiological Catchment Area study. *JAMA* 1990;264(19): 2511–2518.
58. Gerding LB, Labbate LA, Meason MO, et al. Alcohol dependence and hospitalization in schizophrenia. *Schizophr Res* 1999;38(1): 71–75.
59. Kozaric-Kovacic D, Folnegovic-Smalc V, Folnegovic Z. Influence of alcoholism on the prognosis of schizophrenic patients. *J Stud Alcohol* 1995;56(6):622–627.
60. Heila H, Isometsa ET, Henriksson MM, et al. Suicide and schizophrenia: a nationwide psychological autopsy study on age- and sex-specific clinical characteristics of 92 suicide victims with schizophrenia. *Am J Psychiatry* 1997;154(9):1235–1242.
61. Linszen DH, Dingemans PM, Lenior ME. Cannabis abuse and the course of recent onset schizophrenic disorders. *Arch Gen Psychiatry* 1994;51(4):273–279.
62. Levinson I, Galynker II, Rosenthal RN. Methadone withdrawal psychosis. *J Clin Psychiatry* 1995;56(2):73–76.
63. Miotto P, Preti A, Frezza M. Heroin and schizophrenia: subjective responses to abused drugs in dually diagnosed patients. *J Clin Psychopharmacol* 2001;21(1):111–113.

64. Dixon L, Haas G, Weiden PJ, et al. Drug abuse in schizophrenic patients: clinical correlates and reasons for use. *Am J Psychiatry* 1991;148(2):224–230.
65. Schneier FR, Siris SG. A review of psychoactive substance use and abuse in schizophrenia. *J Nerv Ment Dis* 1987;175(11): 641–652.
66. Patkar AA, Alexander RC, Lundy A, et al. Changing patterns of illicit substance use among schizophrenic patients: 1984–96. *Am J Addict* 1999;8(1):65–71.
67. Seibyl JP, Satel SL, Anthony D, et al. Effects of cocaine on hospital course in schizophrenia. *J Nerv Ment Dis* 1993;181:31–37.
68. Sevy S, Kay SR, Opler LA, et al. Significance of cocaine history in schizophrenia. *J Nerv Ment Dis* 1990;178:642–648.
69. Shaner A, Eckman TA, Roberts LJ, et al. Disability income, cocaine use, and repeated hospitalization among schizophrenic cocaine abusers—a government sponsored revolving door? *N Engl J Med* 1995;333(12):777–783.
70. Serper MR, Alpert M, Richardson NA, et al. Clinical effects of recent cocaine use on patients with acute schizophrenia. *Am J Psychiatry* 1995;152(10):1464–1469.
71. Lysaker P, Bell M, Goulet JB, et al. Relationship of positive and negative symptoms to cocaine abuse in schizophrenia. *J Nerv Ment Dis* 1994;182(2):109–112.
72. Miller DD, Kelly MW, Perry PJ, et al. The influence of cigarette smoking on haloperidol pharmacokinetics. *Biol Psychiatry* 1990; 28(6):529–531.
73. Zimmet SV, Strous RD, Burgess ES, et al. Effects of clozapine on substance use in patients with schizophrenia and schizoaffective disorder: a retrospective survey. *J Clin Psychopharmacol* 2000; 20(1):94–98.
74. McCarthy RH. Seizures following smoking cessation in a clozapine responder. *Pharmacopsychiatry* 1994;27(5):210–211.
74a. Barnhill JG, Ciraulo AM, Ciraulo DA, et al. Interactions of importance in chemical dependence. In: Ciraulo DA, Shader RI, Greenblatt DJ, Creelman W, eds. *Drug interactions in psychiatry,* 2nd ed. Baltimore: Williams & Wilkins, 1995:356–398.
75. Tasic M, Simic M, Radic A, et al. Fatal central effects of diazepam potentiated by alcohol and haldol. *Acta Med Legal* 1985;35(1): 185–189.
76. Merab J. Acute dystonic reaction to cocaine. *Am J Med* 1988;84 (3 Pt 1):564.
77. Kumor K, Sherer M, Jaffe J. Haloperidol induced dystonia in cocaine addicts. *Lancet* 1986;2(8519):1341–1342.
78. van Harten PN, van Trier JC, Horwitz EH, et al. Cocaine as a risk factor for neuroleptic induced acute dystonia. *J Clin Psychiatry* 1998;59(3):128–130.
79. Fines RE, Brady WJ, DeBehnke DJ. Cocaine-associated dystonic reaction. *Am J Emerg Med* 1997;15(5):513–515.
80. Cardoso FE, Jankovic J. Cocaine-related movement disorders. *Mov Dis* 1993;8(2):175–178.
81. Hegarty AM, Lipton RB, Merriam AE, et al. Cocaine as a risk factor for acute dystonic reactions. *Neurology* 1991;41(10): 1670–1672.
82. Akpaffiong MJ, Ruiz P. Neuroleptic malignant syndrome: a complication of neuroleptics and cocaine abuse. *Psychiatr Q* 1991; 62(4):299–309.

83. Farren CK, Hameedi FA, Rosen MA, et al. Significant interaction between clozapine and cocaine in cocaine addicts. *Drug Alcohol Depend* 2000;59(2):153–163.

84. Grabowski J, Rhoades H, Silverman P, et al. Risperidone for the treatment of cocaine dependence: randomized, double-blind trial. *J Clin Psychopharmacol* 2000;20(3):305–310.

85. Newton TF, Ling W, Kalechstein AD, et al. Risperidone pretreatment reduces the euphoric effects of experimentally administered cocaine. *Psychiatry Res* 2001;102(3):227–233.

86. Brizer DA, Hartman N, Sweeney J, et al. Effect of methadone plus neuroleptics on treatment resistant chronic paranoid schizophrenia. *Am J Psychiatry* 1985;142(9):1106–1107.

87. Wines JD, Weiss RD. Opioid withdrawal during risperidone treatment. *J Clin Psychopharmacol* 1999;19(3):265–267.

Treating Schizophrenia and Substance Misuse

1. Alcohol user with schizophrenia
   a. Depot neuroleptic in noncompliant patient
   b. Clozapine a good choice
2. Cocaine user with schizophrenia
   a. Increased risk of dystonic reaction with high-potency neuroleptics
   b. Pretreatment with anticholinergic medication advised
   c. Gradual introduction of clozapine a good idea
      i. Caution because of combined effect of cocaine and clozapine decreasing seizure threshold
      ii. Potential for syncopal episode
      iii. Noncompliance likely
   d. Stress need to determine patient's motivations
   e. Schizophrenics with cocaine use are more likely to be paranoid than withdrawn
3. Pregnant cocaine user with schizophrenia
   a. Issues of fetal needs and viability are paramount
   b. Patient's presentation is not that of cocaine psychosis: description given of typical cocaine psychosis
   c. Emphasis placed on risk of depression and suicide in period after stopping cocaine use
4. Heroin user with schizophrenia
   a. Relative rarity of combination of schizophrenia and heroin addiction noted
   b. Stress means of titrating antipsychotic in individual currently on methadone maintenance

TYPICAL PATIENT WITH SCHIZOPHRENIA AND SUBSTANCE ABUSE

CASE 7-1

Chris C. is not unusual among dually diagnosed patients with schizophrenia. He uses both alcohol and marijuana, more of the former because it is cheap, available, and legal, but some of the latter because the people he spends time with smoke it. He is also not uncommon among young people with serious mental illnesses in that he rejects his illness and does not take his medication. Chris is becoming a revolving door patient—in and out of the hospital frequently—with marginal functioning between hospital stays (1,2).

Several ways exist for the treating clinician to approach Chris C. He would benefit from a depot form of medications as his doctors have considered. This would relieve him of the responsibility of daily administration of his medication and give him a chance at stabilization of his condition. For many patients, having to take a pill every day serves as a constant reminder that something is wrong with them. Taking a shot once or twice a month, however, takes away some of the stigma and the responsibility for taking the medication.

Clozapine would also be a good choice, having been demonstrated to decrease consumption of, and craving for, a variety of substances of abuse (3,4). Some degree of reliability is essential, however, for a patient to take clozapine. Further, the patient must be on it for awhile to receive its benefits. Finally, the patient must have a weekly blood test to obtain his medication and Chris C. has not been a cooperative patient to this point. Were he to have an extended hospitalization for some reason, it might be possible to try this. Unfortunately, such an approach is not likely to succeed as long as he is not motivated to change, as appears to be the case. Although the treatment provider needs to try to help motivate Chris C. to change, it is necessary first to get his attention, and so far, this has not happened.

Another possibility is to proceed with the depot form of medication and then slowly introduce clozapine. This, however, can be associated with an increase in use of nicotine, as has been noted (5). Nicotine induces the metabolism of antipsychotics, thus more of the latter must be given. The patient, in turn, is more uncomfortable and smokes more, and so on. Nevertheless, until the patient and the therapist develop some degree of engagement, the revolving door will not be slowed. If Chris C.'s psychosis could be improved somewhat and he could become engaged in treatment, it might then be possible to begin clozapine slowly and concomitantly gradually wean him from the depot neuroleptics. He could then be simultaneously working on his substance use problem.

One approach that is emphatically unacceptable would be to withhold medication because the patient is continuing to use alcohol and other drugs. If Chris C. is willing to take medication because he wants the voices quieted, no justification exists for withholding it.

Engaging Chris C. in treatment is a lengthy process and will take place only over an extended period of time. Professionals providing service for the severely mentally ill will recognize Chris C. as a common and difficult patient with whom a long-term relationship is essential to make progress.

CASE 7-2

Chris C. has been on depot haloperidol for 6 months. His family reports his hygiene is improved and that his auditory hallucinations appear better—at least—they do not hear him talking to himself as much. He continues to drink two or three times a week, although no one is sure how much. Chris sporadically attends a day program. He has not verbalized any goals for being in treatment other than "to get a job." He has had no hospitalizations in that time.

Programs unaccustomed to treating the dually diagnosed patient might consider dismissing Chris C. as "not really wanting to change" or for "noncompliance with treatment." A program catering to the needs of a chronically mentally ill substance misuser would recognize progress and continue to encourage his participation. Chris appears to be drinking only "a couple of times a week," where he had previously been drinking daily. Although his

Table 7-1.   Schizophrenia and alcohol use

Issue	Effects and How Addressed
The "revolving door" patient	Frequent hospitalizations Poor functioning between hospitalizations
Medication noncompliance	Daily administration furthers stigmatization of mental illness Depot neuroleptic can relieve part of the burden
Medication choice	As above, depot neuroleptic can be of benefit Nicotine interaction likely Good safety profile of high potency neuroleptic and alcohol Possibility of naltrexone

attendance at the day program is sporadic, he is attending. Chris C. has actually been able to give a reason for being in the program, although it is not possible to know what "getting a job" can mean for him. Plus, he has had no hospitalizations in 6 months—an improvement from before.

Now might be a good time to try introducing either naltrexone or clozapine to attempt to decrease Chris C.'s alcohol use. In addition, whereas clozapine undoubtedly will help his psychosis, naltrexone may do so as well. The decision regarding which to start depends on how he feels about blood tests and how stable the clinician feels is Chris C.'s attachment to the program. Table 7-1 lists the issues addressed above.

CASE 7-3

Joe L., 26, was diagnosed with schizophrenia at 19 years of age. It was not a surprise when he dropped out of school in the eleventh grade. He had never been a stellar student, and was always such a loner that it was unlikely anyone actually noticed he was no longer there. He drifted through a few low paying jobs, but seemed to have problems keeping them, although he could not quite explain to his parents why. His hygiene deteriorated and eventually he would not leave his room at all without someone prodding him constantly to do so. Finally, it became obvious to everyone around him that he was communicating with someone they could not see, and he was brought to the hospital for help. After his first hospitalization and with his newly acquired disability payments, Joe L. discovered cocaine. With it, he found he could talk to people—even women. He had always been interested in girls, but he had never been able to approach them, let alone ask one out. He had his first sexual experiences under the influence of cocaine. It didn't matter to him if he wound up in jail or in the hospital, cocaine was far superior to anything the doctors or anyone else had come up with to make him feel like he imagined everyone else felt. On the other

hand, family members noticed he seemed to be experiencing a
great deal more depression than he had had before. In addition,
the voices were more common and threatening.

Joe L. is like everyone among individuals with schizophrenia suffering with primarily negative symptoms. The insidious onset,
withdrawn behavior, and lack of social skills are highly characteristic of the disease, as is the energizing symptom relief experienced
with cocaine use (6,7). Some studies indicate that individuals with
schizophrenia and comorbid cocaine use are more likely to suffer
with the paranoid form of the disorder, although whether this is
a result of the cocaine or preceded the onset of use is not clear (7).
Joe L. does not fall into this category of users. Because of his social
withdrawal and the likelihood that he is a rather concrete thinker,
Joe L. is going to be a difficult individual to engage and treat.

If Joe L. is brought to the hospital because of threatening behavior, likely he will receive a shot of a typical neuroleptic medication.
Unfortunately, this may make him more resistant to medication in
the future, as it is increasingly well recognized that cocaine is a significant risk factor for dystonic reactions (8–11). To prevent this
from occurring and improve any chance of Joe L.'s complying with
medication recommendations in the future, the clinician would be
well advised to place him, as well as other cocaine-using individuals with schizophrenia, on prophylactic anticholinergic medication.

It would seem obvious to then follow the same line of reasoning
as with Case 7-2, but some differences should be kept in mind.
Whereas it is true that clozapine does decrease craving for substances of abuse, it is also well known that both cocaine and
clozapine decrease the seizure threshold. The possibility that the
effect might be additive should be kept in mind. In addition, in an
interesting experiment studying the interaction of the two drugs,
Farren et al. (12) administered clozapine to individuals who had
acutely received cocaine. They found that clozapine actually increased serum cocaine levels, although decreased the expected
pleasurable response to the drug. Although no seizures were observed, one subject experienced a near syncopal episode with this
combination. Thus, although clozapine may still be a good choice
for Joe, caution is advised.

As noted in Chapter 6, risperidone too has been shown to decrease
the craving for cocaine in nonpsychotic individuals. This medication
might also be a possibility to decrease the overall effect of the drug.

Joe L. would also be a good candidate to use one of the worksheets
found in Chapter 16, looking at what are his expectations for the
drug versus what the results actually are. For example, it is highly
likely that his hospitalization rate increases with his increased cocaine use. The therapist should determine whether or not Joe L.
likes to be hospitalized. For many patients, hospitalization is a sign
that they have failed. For others, it can mean safety and comfort. If
he does not like hospitalization, his therapist could help Joe L. to plot
the frequency and quantity of cocaine used with the loudness, frequency, and hostility of the voices and the hospitalization rate. This
could demonstrate for Joe L. the relationship between his using and
worsening of symptoms. Dealing with the Joes of the world, always
bear in mind that concrete thinking demands concrete approaches
with information that is personally meaningful to the patient.

Table 7-2. Schizophrenia and cocaine use

Issue	Effects and How Addressed
Onset of schizophrenia	Insidious onset Signs in teens: social withdrawal, low academic achievement
Cocaine effect on schizophrenia	Improvement in negative symptoms Case not typical, as cocaine use is more common in paranoid schizophrenia
Medication	Cocaine increases likelihood of dystonic reactions with neuroleptics Potential risks of cocaine and clozapine interactions Risperidone decreases cocaine craving in nonpsychotic individuals
Other therapeutic issues	Concrete approach to motivation for cocaine use or alternatives to achieving same result

Joe L. was placed on depot haloperidol with some improvement in his symptoms of paranoia and auditory hallucinations. He and his clinician talked for a number of months about what bothered him most about taking medications. His response changed from he "didn't need medication" to he "felt uncomfortable and medication made it difficult to have an erection." With the clinician's assurance he would try to help with the side effects, Joe L. agreed to stay on medication for awhile. At the same time, he saw how much money he was spending on drugs, and listed some thing he could do with that money if he had it available.

Joe L. will likely have periods of exacerbation and remission, but with this concrete and supportive approach, he and others like him will often begin to respond to the requests therapists make of them. Table 7-2 lists the issues addressed above.

CASE 7-4

Everyone says she is pregnant, but Laura S. knows better. It isn't time for her to be pregnant. She only gets pregnant if she wants to be pregnant. And she doesn't want to be pregnant. At 39, or is she 36? She isn't sure if she has ever had a child or not and, if she did, she would have had to leave it at the hospital because it wouldn't be good to her. Of course she knows who the father is, she knows both of them. All of Laura's babies had at least two fathers. She met them in the hospital, but can't remember their names. When Laura presented this information, she did so with an expression of profound sadness and admitted to such feelings. She would shake her head. She can't be pregnant. How could she be pregnant? She smoked crack and that wouldn't be good for a baby, so she can't be pregnant. She only became pregnant when she wanted to be and she didn't want to be. So why did they keep saying she was?

Laura S. is an all too common and undeniably difficult patient to treat. She arrived at the hospital in the company of police, who brought her as a Jane Doe, panhandling in a business area. When asked her name, the visibly pregnant Laura had introduced herself as the Virgin Mary. She willingly signed into the hospital when asked to do so. She complied with most requests, although often had to be asked several times because she was easily confused.

Is she schizophrenic? Bipolar? Schizoaffective? A drug-induced psychosis? It is not clear what the diagnosis is. What is clear is that she is quite psychotic, pregnant, and per the toxicology screen taken at admission, has been using cocaine. She also indicates she is very "sad." This complicated case requires intervention at a number of levels.

An immediate concern is that of the status of the fetus. Regardless of Laura's desires, if she is "visibly pregnant," she is likely past the point at which termination of the pregnancy is legally permissible. In addition, cocaine use has been associated with intrauterine bleeding in the fetus, placental abruption, and other problems, as noted in Chapter 4. It is important to determine the length of gestation and the health of the fetus. If, by chance, the pregnancy is at an age at which an abortion could still be performed, this option could be offered. If, as is more likely, the fetus is viable, close observation and good prenatal care must be arranged immediately.

Concomitantly, as anyone working in a public facility knows, some detective work must be performed. Who is she? She signed in as "Virgin Mary," although she misspelled "vergIn." Looking at the address she gave as "home," it is the address of a homeless shelter. Workers call there and ask vaguely about any pregnant women who might have been living there recently. They are concerned about patient confidentiality, but also about finding friends or family—anyone who might be able to give some history about this patient and her identity. On a Saturday night none of the regular staff will be on duty, and none of the part-timers recognize the description. Come Monday morning, however, the regular staff arrive and recognize the patient as Laura S.

What about her psychosis and "sadness?" Is this simply cocaine induced? It is important for the treating professional to understand that nothing about Laura's presentation is suggestive of a cocaine psychosis. Mitchell and Vierkant (13) report that descriptions of cocaine psychosis date back to the 19th century. Most noteworthy is that animation and paranoia are characteristic of cocaine-induced psychosis. If hallucinations are present, visual and tactile ones are those most common with cocaine, although auditory hallucinations can occur. Laura's emotional withdrawal, her denial of her pregnancy, and her adopting a new identity (the Virgin Mary) are not in any way characteristic of the behavior expected as a result of cocaine alone (13). Laura has a primary psychotic disorder, although it is uncertain exactly which one.

With Laura's "sadness," as always, it is important to probe regarding risk of self-harm. Currently, Laura is very disorganized. In her current state if she were not in the safety of the hospital she would be at great risk of being victimized because of her inability to respond rationally to those around her. In addition,

Laura's inability to correctly interpret environmental cues puts her at risk of accidental trauma, thus posing a further danger to herself. Finally, the clinician must be conscious about suicide and other forms of intentional self-harm.

In terms of her psychosis, some would argue that as long as Laura is in the hospital, willing to permit adequate prenatal care and comply with staff recommendations, no reason is seen to expose the fetus to neuroleptic medication. Others would argue, however, that Laura is not truly competent to make important decisions such as whether to terminate a pregnancy or place a baby for adoption. Therefore, her psychosis must be treated. Medication choices in a case such as this are largely predicated on the needs of the fetus, only taking into the consideration the possibility of drug interactions.

Once Laura's psychosis has resolved, it may be possible to begin to address her cocaine use. While she is acutely ill, no merit is found for attempting to approach the issue. When the subject is raised, the message to be given must be thought out well ahead of time. Laura thinks in a very concrete manner. If Laura is told "cocaine might kill the baby," and Laura does not want the baby anyway, the response may be an increase in cocaine use. Likewise, telling Laura "if you use cocaine, the voices you hear will get louder," and the voices tell her things she likes to hear, the response may also not be the one hoped for. Not all patients dislike the auditory hallucinations.

Laura will need a great deal of hand-holding along with very simple, frequently repeated messages. Examples might be "smoking crack can give you a heart attack" or "makes your asthma worse" (if she has it). It may be necessary to keep her hospitalized through delivery for the safety of the fetus, and only attempt to address the substance use at a later time. The issues addressed above are listed in Table 7-3.

CASE 7-5

Jim, 52, started using heroin in Viet Nam. Most of the guys in his outfit smoked it, so he did too. It was cheap, powerful, and everywhere. Besides, while he was in boot camp, he had noticed a buzzing in his head that almost sounded like someone talking to him. The heroin made it go away, at least for a while. That was years ago. The heroin in the United States was nothing compared to that in Southeast Asia. It didn't stop the voices, which by now were loud and threatening. Besides, he could never seem to get enough to keep from getting sick. One time when he was in the hospital for the voices, they gave him chlorpromazine. He hadn't told them about the heroin, because nobody liked to admit junkies. So Jim was expecting to get very sick in a couple of days. He was pleasantly surprised when the medication quieted the voices down but also took away a lot of the nausea and vomiting he was anticipating. He was still "achy." The muscle cramps and runny nose were there, but they weren't awful. When he was discharged a week later, the voices weren't mocking him. Now on methadone and risperidone, he did not need or want heroin. And for the most part, the voices left him alone.

Table 7-3.   Schizophrenia and pregnancy

Issue	Effects and How Addressed
Pregnancy and psychosis	Determine condition or age of fetus
	Look for intrauterine damage secondary to cocaine use
	Look for viability to help direct decision regarding continuation of pregnancy
	Ability of patient to give informed consent to treat
Patient identification	Issue of breaching patient confidentiality
	Pertinent medical and family history for genetic or pregnancy counseling
Medication issues	Primarily determined by fetal needs
	Avoidance of medications lowering seizure threshold (e.g., clozapine)
Psychiatric issues	Suicide risk
	Presentation not typical of cocaine-induced psychosis
	Risk of victimization because of confusion or inability to comprehend environmental cues
	Issues of ability to give informed consent

Jim is a familiar face among men of his generation. Opiates were used a lot by US troops stationed in Southeast Asia during the Viet Nam era, for all of the reasons listed above. Despite the widespread use overseas, far fewer men continued to use once they returned to the United States. The milieu was different and heroin use was no longer socially acceptable (14), which may be the reason that apparently more opiate-dependent individuals with schizophrenia are in Veterans' Affairs methadone programs in the United States than in other such programs.

Jim also emphasizes the dual role that phenothiazines play therapeutically. Chlorpromazine, for example, was used for its antiemetic properties before its utility as an antipsychotic was discovered. Administering this medication to an individual in heroin withdrawal would be expected to partially suppress the symptoms, as in this case.

The challenge to working with a patient such as Jim is to avoid precipitating withdrawal or a recurrence of psychosis. If the patient is on a stable dose of methadone, introducing or changing neuroleptics must be done carefully. Psychiatric symptoms must be constantly monitored if the patient is on a neuroleptic and methadone is being introduced.

For example, the patient is comfortably on a stable dose of methadone and not using. Further assume the patient is not on a neuroleptic. The case reports cited previously noted the onset of

Table 7-4. Schizophrenia and heroin

Issue	Effects and How Addressed
Opiate use in schizophrenia	Relative rarity of condition
	Antipsychotic property of opiates
Introduction of medication in the methadone maintenance patient	Emphasize need for prolonged titration
	Need for equilibration between dosing changes
	Reduce new medication before increasing methadone

withdrawal symptoms with the introduction of risperidone into such a scenario (15). If risperidone is the agent deemed most appropriate for Jim, and its efficacy and side effect profile are positive, this drug can be administered in a series of very gradual steps. For example, he could be given 1 mg of the antipsychotic at night, and admonished to tell his doctor about any discomfort consistent with withdrawal that he experiences. If the symptoms are significant, the risperidone should be cut in half and no further changes made until the discomfort passes. Once he is comfortable, the medication can be increased again. This pattern can be followed until an effective level of antipsychotic is reached. At each step, a period of adjustment will occur while the two drugs come into equilibrium.

The first reaction to the onset of withdrawal symptoms should be not to increase the methadone. Instead, if the symptoms are more than mild discomfort, the risperidone should be slightly decreased, then advanced more slowly. If the patient's craving for opiates is increasing, a sign that the methadone is no longer achieving an adequate blockade, the risperidone dose should be kept where it is, and the methadone increased.

This is the pattern that should be followed when introducing a psychotropic to a patient on methadone, regardless of what the medication may be. Any other approach results in a chronic imbalance between the drugs so that neither the patient nor the prescribing clinician can determine the source of the patient's discomfort. Table 7-4 lists the issues addressed above.

REFERENCES

1. Haywood TW, Kravitz HM, Grossman LS, et al. Predicting the "revolving door" phenomenon among patients with schizophrenia, schizoaffective, and affective disorders. *Am J Psychiatry* 1995; 152(6):856–861.
2. Birmingham L. Between prison and the community: the 'revolving door psychiatric patient' of the nineties. *Br J Psychiatry* 1999; 174(5):378–379.
3. Buckley P, Thompson P, Way L, et al. Substance abuse among patients with treatment resistant schizophrenia: characteristics and implications for clozapine therapy. *Am J Psychiatry* 1994; 151:385–389.

4. Zimmet SV, Strous RD, Burgess ES, et al. Effects of clozapine on substance use in patients with schizophrenia and schizoaffective disorder: a retrospective survey. *J Clin Psychopharmacol* 2000; 20(1):94–98.
5. Dalack GW, Healy DJ, Meador-Woodruff JH. Nicotine dependence in schizophrenia: clinical phenomena and laboratory findings. *Am J Psychiatry* 1998;155(11):1490–1501.
6. Serper MR, Alpert M, Richardson NA, et al. Clinical effects of recent cocaine use on patients with acute schizophrenia. *Am J Psychiatry* 1995;152(10):1464–1469.
7. Lysaker P, Bell M, Goulet JB, et al. Relationship of positive and negative symptoms to cocaine abuse in schizophrenia. *J Nerv Ment Dis* 1994;182(2):109–112.
8. van Harten PN, van Trier JC, Horwitz EH, et al. Cocaine as a risk factor for neuroleptic induced acute dystonia. *J Clin Psychiatry* 1998;59(3):128–130.
9. Hegarty AM, Lipton RB, Merriam AE, et al. Cocaine as a risk factor for acute dystonic reactions. *Neurology* 1991;41(10):1670–1672.
10. Fines RE, Brady WJ, DeBehnke DJ. Cocaine-associated dystonic reaction. *Am J Emerg Med* 1997;15(5):513–515.
11. Cardoso FE, Jankovic J. Cocaine-related movement disorders. *Mov Disord* 1993;8(2):175–178.
12. Farren CK, Hameedi FA, Rosen MA, et al. Significant interaction between clozapine and cocaine in cocaine addicts. *Drug Alcohol Depend* 2000;59(2):153–163.
13. Mitchell J, Vierkant AD. Delusions and hallucinations of cocaine and paranoid schizophrenics: a comparative study. *J Psychol* 1991;125(3):301–311.
14. Robins LN, Helzer JE, Davis DH. Narcotic use in southeast Asia and afterward. An interview study of 898 Vietnam returnees. *Arch Gen Psychiatry* 1975;32(8):955–961.
15. Wines JD, Weiss RD. Opioid withdrawal during risperidone treatment. *J Clin Psychopharmacol* 1999;19(3):265–267.

8

Bipolar Disorder and Substance Misuse

1. Bipolar disorder not a single entity
   a. Occurs on a continuum: three subtypes
   b. Depending on definition, occurs in 1% to 6% of population
2. Hallmark is alteration in mood
   a. Moods can occur in pure depression, mania, or mixed forms
   b. Moods do not need to alternate between first one then the other; one can predominate
3. Demographics
   a. Onset typically in adolescence or young adulthood
   b. Male:female occurrence is same
   c. Mixed type more common in females
   d. Childhood onset more common in males
4. Etiology: genetic and environmental influences
5. Medication response
   a. Mood stabilizers of most importance: response rate 40% to 70%
   b. Suicide risk decreased with use of these agents, especially lithium, with risk increasing with drug discontinuation
6. Comorbidity
   a. Highest rate of comorbidity of the major psychiatric disorders
   b. Chances of comorbidity increase with adolescent onset and mixed mania
   c. Alcohol use and stimulant use both extremely common here and in cultures where substance use not usual
   d. Substance misuse increases likelihood of poor compliance and of suicide
7. Specific substances and bipolar disorder
   a. Nicotine: use high, double that of normal population
   b. Alcohol: misuse of this substance about six times that of normal population; presence increases suicide risk
   c. Marijuana: effect of use equivocal: can have calming effect or can induce psychosis
   d. Opioids: effect of use equivocal: evidence of improvement of both mania and depression with opioids
   e. Cocaine: appears to induce mania
8. Medication effects of substances of abuse
   a. Bipolar disorder and comorbidity predict poor response to lithium
   b. Valproic acid preferred medication in this population
   c. Other anticonvulsants can also be of benefit

BACKGROUND

Many writers have noted the fine line between genius and madness. When this observation is made, it is bipolar illness that is described because of its condition of hypomania in which the individual has a greatly increased capacity for activity with a decreased need for sleep. Lord Byron was described by a contemporary as "mad," but the observer went on to dispel the idea that this was somehow unique, saying ". . . as are all poets" (1). Vincent van Gogh produced most of his most famous works during a single manic episode. Both of these individuals plus others including Honoré de Balzac, Robert Schumann, Ernest Hemingway, and Virginia Woolf are believed to have had bipolar illness (1).

The term "bipolar disorder" does not refer to a single entity, but rather to a continuum of disorders consisting of several subtypes: bipolar I, bipolar II, and cyclothymia. Bipolar disorder emphasizes the polar extremes of mood the sufferer exhibits: moods including mania, hypomania, depression, and mixed affect. Most commonly, bipolar disorder is said to occur in approximately 1% of the population. If bipolar II and cyclothymia are included in the tally, bipolar spectrum disorder may afflict up to 6% of adults (2).

Manic episodes can occur suddenly or after a more prolonged and insidious onset. Regardless of the pattern of onset, full-blown mania, with its characteristics of severely impaired judgment and impulsivity, is disabling and can be destructive to individuals and to those around them.

On the opposite end of the spectrum is potentially life-threatening depression. Risk of suicide in bipolar disorder is substantial— more than ten times that of the general population. Most successful suicides occur during the depressed phase of the disorder (2–7).

Mixed mania has features of both depression and mania. Typically, the condition is characterized by heightened activity but depressed mood. The existence of this phenomenon was recognized by Kraepelin more than 75 years ago (8). It occurs more commonly in women and in those with onset in adolescence (9,10). Both suicidal ideation and suicide attempts are found in greater frequency among individuals with mixed mania than with pure mania (11,12).

For many years, the literature stressed the cyclical nature of manic versus depressed states. A popularly held belief was that manic episodes occurred in the spring, depressed episodes in fall. Whereas some evidence suggests that hospitalization rates for first episode depression in bipolar illness may be slightly increased in the fall of the year, data from various countries generally fail to otherwise support the idea of a seasonal variation to admissions for mania and depression (13–16). It is not known, however, if a seasonal variation exists for mood shifts of lesser intensity not requiring hospitalization. Individuals with bipolar disorder do not necessarily have alternating periods of mania followed by depression. Rather, they may have repeated episodes of one type of affective state before eventually changing to another (17).

ONSET

Most cases of bipolar disorder have their onset in late adolescence and early adulthood. A small but significant number of cases are recognized in preadolescent children as well. Although bipolar disorder occurs in men and women at the same rate, the variant of the condition showing onset in childhood tends to occur more often in boys. Studies show that approximately one third of children with major depression will later be diagnosed with bipolar disorder. Juvenile onset predicts a more malignant course of bipolar disorder, and moods are more likely to be mixed in nature (18,19) (Table 8-1).

ETIOLOGY

As with schizophrenia, it appears that both environmental and genetic factors play a role in the genesis of bipolar disorder. Some indications are that more people diagnosed with bipolar disorder

**Table 8-1.   Comparison: dually diagnosed
vs. not dually diagnosed bipolar**

	Bipolar Disorder Alone	Dually Diagnosed Bipolar Disorder
Age at diagnosis	Later onset	Younger onset, male = risk factor
Family history	Increased rate of affective disorders	Increased rate of affective disorders and of substance use disorders
Risk of suicide	Increased over general population	Increase over bipolar alone and well above general population
Risk of violence	Greater than normal population	Much increased above normal population and above bipolar disorder alone
Rate of hospitalization	Baseline for disorder	Increases hospitalization rate
Medication compliance	+/– with lithium; better with depakote	Poor in general
Long-term outcome	Fair	Poorer
Incidence of mixed mania	More common in females	Increased and less responsive to lithium
Episodes of mania and depression	Same	Same

are born in winter and early spring than any other time of the year, raising questions of an infectious or climatic contribution to its onset (20,21) (Table 8-1).

Numerous studies have demonstrated that bipolar disorder runs in families. Other psychiatric disorders occur within families of individuals with bipolar disorder as well. For example, both unipolar depression and schizoaffective disorder (but not schizophrenia) occur more frequently among first-degree relatives of individuals with bipolar disorder (22). Bipolar offspring of individuals with bipolar illness tend to show signs of the disorder at an earlier age than do those without first-degree relatives with the diagnosis (23). In addition, those with a family history of bipolar disorder tend to have more and more frequent episodes of mania and depression (24). Further data supporting the genetic basis of bipolar disorder come from studies demonstrating changes at the level of chromosome four among members of families in which the disorder commonly occurs (25).

MEDICATION RESPONSE

Response rates to medication among individuals with bipolar disorder range from 40% to 70%, with recovery from manic and mixed episodes highly dependent on compliance with medication (26). Although antipsychotics and antidepressants provide relief of symptoms of mania and depression, respectively, the gold standard of treatment of bipolar disorder is use of mood stabilizers, including lithium, valproic acid, and carbamazepine, among others. Treatment with such agents is associated with a decreased risk of suicide. Discontinuation, on the other hand, especially abrupt discontinuation, results in return of affective symptoms among two thirds of patients as well as a substantial increase in suicidal acts (27–29) (Table 8-1).

COMORBIDITY

Estimates are that bipolar illness is associated with the highest incidence of comorbid substance misuse of all the major psychiatric disorders (26,30,31). Comorbidity rates of up to 75% are found in the literature (24,32) (Table 8-2). The chances of having comorbid bipolar and substance use disorders increase with adolescent onset of illness, mixed mania, and a family history of substance misuse (33,34). Childhood onset bipolar illness, however, does not increase the risk for substance abuse that characterizes adolescent onset (35).

Even in cultures where alcohol use is not common, alcohol is widely abused among individuals with bipolar disorder (36,37). Researchers in the United States have found stimulant abuse is also excessive in this population (32). Both men and women with bipolar disorder are at high risk of substance use disorders. Reports vary whether men or women are more susceptible to such (32,34,38–40).

A substance use disorder worsens the prognosis for the patient with bipolar disorder. Whereas the number of episodes of mania and depression may be similar among those with and without comorbid conditions, those with characteristically have poorer treatment compliance, increased risk of aggression, and are hospitalized more often than are those without comorbid conditions (Table 8-3). In addition, the risk of suicide is increased among persons with bipolar and substance use disorders (41–43).

BIPOLAR DISORDER AND NICOTINE

The rate of tobacco use among individuals with bipolar disorder is higher than that of the general population (44), and the most thought-disordered individuals use the most nicotine (45). Studies both in the United States and abroad give a prevalence

Table 8-2.   Bipolar disorder and comorbidity

Highest incidence of comorbidity ≈75%
Alcohol use common, even in cultures where its use is uncommon
Stimulant use common
Predictive of poor compliance

Table 8-3. Substance use and bipolar disorder

Substance	Incidence with Bipolar Disorder	Effect on Treatment	Medication Effects	Other Issues
Nicotine	↑↑Amount used ≅ psychosis			
Alcohol	↑↑↑ with bipolar disorder	↑ Risk of suicide	Valproic acid was useful in one small study with no increase in liver function tests; lithium relatively less effective	Females show increased anxiety and depression
Cannabis	No data	May relieve both manic and depressive symptoms	Possible interaction with lithium results in lithium toxicity	Possibly induces psychosis
Opioids	No data	Both antimanic and antidepressant effects?	Carbamazepine decreases methadone levels; not affected by valproic acid	Issue of tolerance limits usefulness as treatment of affective disorder
Psychostimulants	Increased use with bipolar disorder; greater in manic state	↓ Compliance with recommendations	Decreased likelihood of lithium response	

rate of nicotine use among individuals with bipolar disorder to be approximately double that of the general population, and close to that of individuals with schizophrenia (46,47). As noted elsewhere, evidence shows a positive effect of nicotine on mood in other disorders. Whether such effects occur specifically with bipolar disorder is not known.

BIPOLAR DISORDER AND ALCOHOL

Alcohol use disorders are substantially more prevalent among individuals with bipolar disorder than among the general population. According to one group, it is more than six times that of the normal population (48). Women with bipolar disorder and alcohol dependence have more depression and anxiety than either men with such comorbid conditions or women with bipolar disorder only (49). The presence of alcohol substantially increases the risk of suicide (50–52).

CASE 8-1

The patient, Martin T., 35 years of age, is a veteran of the Gulf War who suffered his first manic episode while serving in the Middle East at the end of that conflict. He spent much of 1 year, first in a military hospital in Germany, then in a stateside facility for further rehabilitation. Over the last decade he has been incarcerated and hospitalized numerous times, largely because of stopping his lithium and resuming his heavy alcohol use. During periods of mania, he has been known to drink in excess of two fifths of vodka per day. The patient indicates he wants to alter the downward path his life has taken, but does not feel able to stop his drinking.

BIPOLAR DISORDER AND MARIJUANA

Anecdotal reports suggest that marijuana can have some mood stabilizing effects in relieving both mania and depression in some patients with bipolar disorder (53). The literature is also full of reports, however, of psychotic reactions among individuals without histories of psychosis when smoking high potency cannabis in south Asian countries (54–59).

BIPOLAR DISORDER AND OPIOIDS

It has long been suggested that opioids possess antidepressant effects, but the addictive potential of all members of the opioid family limits their use for this purpose. Some researchers, however, have further identified antimanic effects of opioid agents. Trials of methadone, for example, have demonstrated that this agent results in reduction in "euphoria and grandiosity" in acutely manic individuals. Once again, however, the issues of tolerance and dependence have rendered this line of research less desirable (60).

BIPOLAR DISORDER AND PSYCHOSTIMULANTS

Use of psychostimulants increases the rate of hospitalization among those with bipolar disorder and decreases the likelihood of compliance with medication as well as other recommendations

(61,62). The use of psychostimulants is disproportionately associated with cyclothymia, although cause and effect is not clear (63). Contrary to the idea that addicted individuals might be self-medicating an underlying problem, it appears cocaine users with bipolar illness are further boosting their hypomania into full-blown mania. Likewise, studies show cocaine use is more common during manic episodes than is alcohol use.

MEDICATION EFFECTS

Issues regarding substances of abuse as they affect antidepressants and antipsychotics are discussed in the chapters on depression and schizophrenia, respectively. In general, it should be noted that patients with bipolar disorder who abuse alcohol and other substances do not tend to respond well to lithium. In fact, lithium may cause unforeseen problems in this population. In their comprehensive review of the literature, Sarid-Segal et al. (64) elaborate on a 1981 case of lithium toxicity that occurred when a patient began to use marijuana. Instead, such patients may demonstrate a better response with anticonvulsant mood stabilizers (65). This may reflect the fact that substance-abusing individuals with bipolar disorder are more susceptible to experiencing mixed than pure affective states (38).

Given the risk of liver disease in this population from hepatitis and alcohol-related damage, it is important to know which anticonvulsant to use. Despite concerns about hepatotoxicity and pancreatitis, in a very small open label trial, Brady et al. found that valproate was effective in relieving manic symptoms in substance-abusing individuals with bipolar disorder and did not produce liver abnormalities (66). Carbamazepine can cause problems in opioid-dependent individuals with bipolar disorder in that it can lower methadone levels, an effect that valproic acid does not possess (67).

El-Mallakh (68) showed methylphenidate to be safe and effective in decreasing the depression in depressed patients with bipolar disorder. A problem with this, however, is that the suggestion has been made that methylphenidate administration to cocaine users could result in increased craving for, and use of, cocaine (69). Although this has not been found to be the case in combined trials, numerous reports appear in the literature of the sale and misuse of this substance (70–74). Therefore, prescribing methylphenidate to individuals already known to abuse substances cannot be recommended.

REFERENCES

1. Jamison KR. *Touched with fire: manic depressive illness and the artistic temperament.* New York: The Free Press, 1993.
2. Angst J, Preisig M. Outcome of a clinical cohort of unipolar, bipolar, and schizoaffective patients: results of a prospective study from 1959–1985. *Schwiez Archives of Neurology and Psychiatry* 1995;146(1):17–23.
3. Isometsa ET, Henriksson MM, Aro HM, et al. Suicide in bipolar disorder in Finland. *Am J Psychiatry* 1994;151(7):1020–1024.
4. Nordstrom P, Asberg M, Aberg-Wistedt A, et al. Attempted suicide predicts suicide risk in mood disorders. *Acta Psychiatr Scand* 1995;92(5):345–350.

5. Strakowski SM, DelBello MP. The co-occurrence of bipolar and substance use disorders. *Clin Psychol Rev* 2000;20(2):191–206.
6. Simpson SG, Jamison KR. The risk of suicide in patients with bipolar disorder. *J Clin Psychiatry* 1999;60(Suppl 2):53–56.
7. Tondo L, Baldesarini RJ, Hennen J, et al. Suicide attempts in major affective disorder patients with comorbid substance use disorders. *J Clin Psychiatry* 1999;60(Suppl 2):63–69.
8. Freeman MP, McElroy SL. Clinical picture and etiologic models of mixed states. In: Agiskal HS, ed. *Bipolarity: beyond classic mania,* Vol. 22. Philadelphia: WB Saunders, 1999:535–546.
9. Coryell W, Endicott J, Keller M. Rapid cycling affective disorder: demographics, diagnosis, family history, and course. *Arch Gen Psychiatry* 1992;49:126–131.
10. Wehr TA, Sack DA, Rosenthal NE, et al. Rapid cycling affective disorder: contributing factors and treatment responses in 51 patients. *Am J Psychiatry* 1988;145:179–184.
11. Strakowski SM, McElroy SL, Keck PE, et al. Suicidality among patients with mixed and manic bipolar disorder. *Am J Psychiatry* 1996;153:674–676.
12. Dilsaver SC, Chen YW, Swann AC, et al. Suicidality in patients with pure and depressive mania. *Am J Psychiatry* 1994;151: 1312–1314.
13. Partonen T, Lonnqvist J. Seasonal variation in bipolar disorder. *Br J Psychiatry* 1996;169(5):641–646.
14. Whitney DK, Sharma V, Kueneman K. Seasonality of manic depressive illness in Canada. *J Affect Disord* 1999;55(2–3):99–105.
15. Silverstone T, Romans S, Hunt N, et al. Is there a seasonal pattern of relapse in bipolar affective disorders? A dual Northern and Southern Hemisphere cohort study. *Br J Psychiatry* 1995;167(1): 58–60.
16. Hunt N, Sayer H, Silverstone T. Season and manic relapse. *Acta Psychiatr Scand* 1992;85(2):123–126.
17. Akiskal HS. The clinical necessity of a return to Kraepelin's broad schema of manic depression. In: Akiskal HS, ed. *Bipolarity: beyond classic mania,* Vol. 22. Philadelphia: WB Saunders, 1999:xi.
18. Todd RD, Geller B, Neuman R, et al. Increased prevalence of alcoholism in relatives of depressed and bipolar children. *J Am Acad Child Adolesc Psychiatry* 1996;35(6):716–724.
19. Carlson GA, Bromet EJ, Sievers S. Phenomenology and outcome of subjects with early—and adult onset psychotic mania. *Am J Psychiatry* 2000;571(2):213–219.
20. Torrey EF, Miller J, Rawlings R, et al. Seasonality of birth in schizophrenia and bipolar disorder: a review of the literature. *Schizophr Res* 1997;28(1):1–38.
21. Boyd JH, Pulver AE, Stewart W. Season of birth: schizophrenia and bipolar disorder. *Schizophr Bull* 1986;12(2):173–186.
22. Kendler KS, McGuire M, Gruenberg AM, et al. The Roscommon Family Study. IV. Affective illness, anxiety disorders, and alcoholism in relatives. *Arch Gen Psychiatry* 1993;50(12):952–960.
23. Grigoroiu-Serbanescu M, Wickramaratne PJ, Hodge SE, et al. Genetic anticipation and imprinting in bipolar I illness. *Br J Psychiatry* 1997;170:162–166.
24. Winokur G, Coryell W, Akiskal H, et al. Manic depressive (bipolar) disorder: the course in light of a prospective ten year follow up of 131 patients. *Acta Psychiatr Scand* 1994;89(2):102–110.

25. Kennedy JL, Basile VS, Macciardi FM. Chromosome 4 workshop summary: Sixth World congress on psychiatric genetics, Bonn, Germany. *Am J Med Genet* 1999;88(3):224–248.
26. Goldberg JF, Harrow M. Poor outcome bipolar disorders. In: Goldberg JF, Harrow M, eds. *Bipolar disorders: clinical course and outcome.* Washington, DC: American Psychiatric Press, 1999.
27. Tondo L, Baldesarini RJ, Hennen J, et al. Lithium treatment and risk of suicidal behavior in bipolar disorder patients. *J Clin Psychiatry* 1998;59(8):405–414.
28. Tondo L, Hennen J, Baldessarini RJ. Lower suicide risk with long-term lithium treatment in major affective illness: a meta-analysis. *Acta Psychiatr Scand* 2001;104(3):163–172.
29. Baldessarini RJ, Tondo L, Hennen J. Effects of lithium treatment and its discontinuation on suicidal behavior in bipolar manic-depressive disorders. *J Clin Psychiatry* 1999;60(Suppl 2): 77–84.
30. Winokur G, Coryell W, Akiskal H, et al. Alcoholism in manic depressive (bipolar) illness; familial illness, course of illness, and the primary-secondary distinction. *Am J Psychiatry* 1995;152(3): 365–372.
31. Winokur G, Coryell W, Endicott J, et al. Familial alcoholism in manic depressive (bipolar) disease. *Am J Med Genet* 1996;67(2): 197–201.
32. Tohen M, Zarate CAJ. Bipolar disorder and comorbid substance use disorder. In: Goldberg JF, Harrow M, eds. *Bipolar disorders: clinical course and outcome.* Washington, DC: American Psychiatric Press, 1999:171–184.
33. Mueser KT, Yarnold PR, Bellack AS. Diagnostic and demographic correlates of substance abuse in schizophrenia and major affective disorder. *Acta Psychiatr Scand* 1992;85(1):48–55.
34. Tohen M, Greenfield SF, Weiss RD, et al. The effect of comorbid substance use disorders on the course of bipolar disorder: a review. *Harv Rev Psychiatry* 1998;6(3):133–141.
35. Wilens TE, Biederman J, Millstein RB, et al. Risk for substance use disorders in youths with child and adolescent onset bipolar disorder. *J Am Acad Child Adolesc Psychiatry* 1999;38(6): 680–685.
36. Tsai SY, Chen CC, Yeh EK. Alcohol problems and long-term psychosocial outcome in Chinese patients with bipolar disorder. *J Affect Disord* 1997;46(2):143–150.
37. Lin CC, Bai YM, Hu PG, et al. Substance use disorders among inpatients with bipolar disorder and major depressive disorder in a general hospital. *Gen Hosp Psychiatry* 1998;20(2):98–101.
38. Goldberg JF, Garno JL, Leon AC, et al. A history of substance abuse complicates remission from acute mania in bipolar disorder. *J Clin Psychiatry* 1999;60(11):733–740.
39. Lambert MT, Griffith JM, Hendrickse W. Characteristics of patients with substance abuse diagnoses on a general psychiatry unit in a VA Medical Center. *Psychiatr Serv* 1996;47(10):1104–1107.
40. Winokur G, Turvey C, Akiskal H, et al. Alcoholism and drug abuse in three groups: bipolar I, unipolars, and their acquaintances. *J Affect Disord* 1998;50(2–3):81–89.
41. Havassy BE, Arns PG. Relationship of cocaine and other substance dependence to well-being of high-risk psychiatric patients. *Psychiatr Serv* 1998;49(7):935–940.

42. Kessing LV. The effect of comorbid alcoholism on recurrence in affective disorder: a case register study. *J Affect Disord* 1999;53(1): 49–55.
43. Sonne SC, Brady KT, Morton WA. Substance abuse and bipolar affective disorder. *J Nerv Ment Dis* 1994;182(6):349–352.
44. Gonzalez-Pinto A, Gutierrez M, Ezcurra J, et al. Tobacco smoking and bipolar disorder. *J Clin Psychiatry* 1998;59(5):225–228.
45. Corvin A, O'Mahony E, O'Regan M, et al. Cigarette smoking and psychotic symptoms in bipolar affective disorder. *Br J Psychiatry* 2001;179:35–38.
46. Itkin O, Nemets B, Einat H. Smoking habits in bipolar and schizophrenic outpatients in southern Israel. *J Clin Psychiatry* 2001; 62(4):269–272.
47. Lasser K, Boyd JW, Woolhandler S, et al. Smoking and mental illness: a population based prevalence study. *JAMA 2000;* 284(20): 2606–2610.
48. Helzer J, Pryzbeck T. The co-occurrence of alcoholism with other psychiatric disorders in the general population and its impact on treatment. *J Stud Alcohol* 1988;49:219–224.
49. Salloum IM, Cornelius JR, Mezzich JE, et al. Characterizing female bipolar alcoholic patients presenting for initial evaluation. *Addict Behav* 2001;26(3):341–348.
50. Goldberg JF, Garno JL, Portera L, et al. Correlates of suicidal ideation in dysphoric mania. *J Affect Disord* 1999;56(1):75–81.
51. Verstergaard P, Aagaard J. Five-year mortality in lithium treated manic depressive patients. *J Affect Disord* 1991;21(1):33–38.
52. Potash JB, Kane HS, Chiu YF, et al. Attempted suicide and alcoholism in bipolar disorder: clinical and familial relationships. *Am J Psychiatry* 2000;157(12):2048–2050.
53. Grinspoon L, Bakalar JB. The use of cannabis as a mood stabilizer in bipolar disorder: anecdotal evidence and the need for clinical research. *J Psychoactive Drugs* 1998;30(2):171–177.
54. Chopra GS, Smith JW. Psychotic reactions following cannabis use in east Indians. *Arch Gen Psychiatry* 1974;30:24–27.
55. Chaudry HR, Moss HB, Bashir A, et al. Cannabis psychosis following bhang ingestion. *British Journal of Addiction* 1991;86(9): 1075–1081.
56. Spencer J. Cannabis psychosis in young psychiatric patients. *British Journal of Addiction* 1987;82(10):1155.
57. Kroll P. Psychoses associated with marijuana use in Thailand. *J Nerv Ment Dis* 1975;161(3):149–156.
58. Thacore VR. Bhang psychosis. *Br J Psychiatry* 1973;123(573): 225–229.
59. Bernhardson G, Gunne LM. Forty-six cases of psychosis in cannabis abusers. *International Journal of Addictions* 1972;7(1):9–16.
60. Gold MS, Pottash AC, Sweeney D, et al. Antimanic, antidepressant, and antipanic effects of opiates: clinical, neuroanatomical, and biochemical evidence. *Ann NY Acad Sci* 1982;398:140–150.
61. Havassy BE, Arns PG. Relationship of cocaine and other substance dependence to well being of high risk psychiatric patients. *Psychiatr Serv* 1998;49(7):935–940.
62. Wolpe PR, Gorton G, Serota R, et al. Predicting compliance of dual diagnosis inpatients with aftercare treatment. *Hospital and Community Psychiatry* 1993;44(1):45–49.
63. Mirin SM, Weiss RD, Griffin ML, et al. Psychopathology in drug abusers and their families. *Compr Psychiatry* 1991;32(1):36–51.

64. Sarid-Segal O, Creelman WL, Ciraulo DA, et al. Lithium. In: Ciraulo DA, Shader RI, Greenblatt DJ, et al., eds. *Drug interactions in psychiatry*. Baltimore: Williams & Wilkins, 1995: 175–213.
65. Nunes EV, McGrath PJ, Wager S, et al. Lithium treatment for cocaine abusers with bipolar spectrum disorders. *Am J Psychiatry* 1990;147(5):655–657.
66. Brady KT, Sonne SC, Anton R, et al. Valproate in the treatment of acute bipolar affective episodes complicated by substance abuse: a pilot study. *J Clin Psychiatry* 1995;56(3):118–121.
67. Ciraulo DA, Shader RI, Greenblatt DJ, et al., eds. *Drug interactions in psychiatry*. Baltimore: Williams & Wilkins, 1995.
68. El-Mallakh RS. An open study of methylphenidate in bipolar depression. *Bipolar Disord* 2000;2(1):56–59.
69. Gawin FH, Riordan C, Kleber H. Methylphenidate treatment of cocaine abusers without attention deficit disorder: a negative report. *Am J Drug Alcohol Abuse* 1985;11:193–197.
70. Grabowski J, Roache JD, Schmitz JM, et al. Replacement medication for cocaine dependence: methylphenidate. *J Clin Psychopharmacol* 1997;17(6):485–488.
71. Parran TV, Jasinski DR. Intravenous methylphenidate abuse: prototype for prescription drug abuse. *Arch Intern Med* 1991;151:781–783.
72. Wolf J, Fein A, Fehrenbacher L. Eosinophilic syndrome with methylphenidate abuse. *Ann Intern Med* 1978;89:224–225.
73. Spensley J, Rockwell DA. Psychosis during methylphenidate abuse. *N Engl J Med* 1972;286:880–881.
74. Hayashi RJ, Gill MA, Kern JW, et al. Characteristics of eosinophilia in a series of intravenous methylphenidate abusers. *Drug Intelligence & Clinical Pharmacy* 1980;14:189–192.

Treatment of Bipolar Disorder and Substance Misuse

1. The noncompliant patient with comorbid bipolar disorder and alcohol misuse
    a. Lithium is poor choice for mood stabilizer; valproic acid or another anticonvulsant preferred
    b. Clozapine beneficial in treatment-refractory bipolar disorder
    c. Clozapine decreases appetite for alcohol
    d. Tricyclic antidepressant should be avoided because of potential for interaction with alcohol and for inducing rapid cycling mania
    e. Addressing use of alcohol
        i.   Offer naltrexone for decreasing alcohol consumption
        ii. Avoid disulfiram
        iii. Other new agents may be available soon
2. Patient with comorbid marijuana use and bipolar disorder
    a. Typical for marijuana and alcohol use to co-occur
    b. Lack of structure and socialization mitigate against patient being abstinent
    c. Avoidance of disulfiram, but additional problem of marijuana and disulfiram interaction
3. Comorbid bipolar disorder and cocaine use
    a. Establish pattern of use
    b. Depressive symptoms require medication: serotonin reuptake inhibitor
    c. Identifying causes of noncompliance an issue
    d. Suggestions made for addressing weight gain associated with medications

Clinicians working in the public sector will recognize Case 8-1 with bipolar disorder and substance misuse as a common visitor to general hospital emergency rooms. This patient is also a very expensive individual to treat, being a "revolving door" patient (1–3). The revolving door patient, as discussed elsewhere, is one who is frequently in and out of the hospital, typically has comorbid psychotic and substance use disorders, and is noncompliant with medications. Although this patient is very difficult to treat, it does not mean treatment is impossible. It simply means that the treatment provider must take much time in engaging the patient, be creative in the approach, and help the patient find a motivation for change.

If the resources exist to do so, containing the patient in the hospital for a period of time for drying out and observation would be helpful. Ideally, this would be followed by case management services and day hospital participation in order to help the patient structure his or her time. If containment is not possible, helping the patient establish some degree of structure is essential. Many programs and providers encourage such patients to show up at the same time and place every day or several days per week for group therapy or activities and socialization. The intent is to reduce the patient's idle time and isolation, and to begin to establish concrete expectations.

It would also be helpful to know what the patient wants for him- or herself—now and for the future. For example, does the patient want to stay out of the hospital and out of jail? For many patients, hospitalization is a failure. For others, however, it is a chance to be taken care of, to socialize, or to feel safe and warm and have their dependency needs met. Likewise, some patients want to avoid jail at all costs, whereas others do not mind it; it is a place to be in out of the weather, to be warm, and to be fed. Still other patients, perhaps a patient who has verbalized the belief that change may not be possible, wants help and a different life, but fears to hope that this can be accomplished. Whereas all patients require encouragement and support, the patient who feels change is not possible needs help to avoid discouragement and hopelessness. It must also be borne in mind that patients with bipolar illness are at increased risk of suicide, and those with comorbid substance misuse are at a higher risk still (4).

Next is the issue of medication. As stated, lithium is generally ineffective in dually diagnosed patients—even ones who, unlike patient 8-1, take it (5,6). This patient needs to be on a different mood stabilizer. It is possible that just helping to control the patient's affect will improve the chances of reducing the number of returns to the hospital. Valproic acid, with careful monitoring of liver functions and amylase, is a good choice. Likewise, carbamazepine, with monitoring of bone marrow functioning, could be initiated. Other promising agents are gabapentin and lamotrigine, although neither currently has the body of evidence to support its usefulness that the previous two medications have (7–9). If, however, their benefit is proved, lamotrigine and gabapentin may be preferable for the treatment of bipolar patients with comorbid alcohol dependence because of their safety profile and the fact that it is not necessary to monitor blood levels (9).

In the event that an antipsychotic is needed, atypical antipsychotics are better choices than the typical agents, which can actually increase the use of some substances, as discussed in Chapter 6 (10). Clozapine, for example, has proved to be beneficial in the treatment of refractory bipolar illness (11–14). A significant problem with using clozapine in this population, however, is seeing that the patient obtains the blood test necessary to receive the medication. If this logistic problem can be overcome, clozapine has a significant advantage over other antipsychotics. It has been shown to decrease the use of alcohol, cocaine, and nicotine among individuals with schizophrenia and schizoaffective disorder. Although studies specifically aimed at bipolar disorder are lacking, it is reasonable to believe clozapine will have the same effect with individuals with comorbid bipolar disorder and substance misuse (10,15).

Finally, is the issue of an antidepressant. A significant body of evidence suggests that tricyclic antidepressants (TCA) induce rapid cycling (16). In addition, given the potential for alcohol–medication interactions and the increased risk of suicide in comorbid bipolar disorder and alcohol misuse, tricyclics should be used only with great caution. If, because of cost or other constraints, a TCA is used in this case, very limited quantities should be made available to the patient at any one time. More data are available on the serotonin reuptake inhibitors (SSRI) in the treatment of bipolar disorder and their interactions with alcohol than for all the newer antidepressants, including nefazodone, mirtazapine, and venflavaxine, combined. Thus, at this point, the safest route is to recommend an SSRI until more is known about these other agents.

The patient's alcohol use should now be addressed. Assuming the patient does not need to be detoxified from this drug, an issue addressed in Chapter 5, it would be helpful to have a discussion about the patient's desire for alcohol. Does the patient crave it? That is, do the commercials and billboards about beer and spirits trigger an intense longing for a drink? If so, the patient might benefit from using naltrexone. Naltrexone appears to help some alcohol abusers curb their craving for alcohol and reduce their alcohol consumption, although it does not work for everyone (17,18). In addition, over the last 10 years, a number of studies have evaluated naltrexone for treating psychosis. The results, at best, have been equivocal. However, it does not appear that this medication causes any worsening of psychotic symptoms (19–21). Thus, a trial of this drug might help alcohol-craving patients with bipolar illness curb their appetite for the drug of choice. Likewise acamprosate, the likely to be legalized anticraving drug, might be tried for the patient craving alcohol. Studies are currently underway with psychiatrically impaired populations, to assess the effect of this medication on such individuals.

Disulfiram (Antabuse, Wyeth-Ayerst, Philadelphia, PA), as discussed elsewhere, is a medication used to induce an aversive reaction when alcohol is ingested. Ample evidence exists to suggest that this medication should not be used in individuals with a tendency to psychosis, or used only with extreme caution. Reports spanning more than two decades suggest that individuals with preexisting psychiatric disturbances are susceptible to psychotic reactions when exposed to disulfiram (22–24).

If a patient, in fact, wants to change his or her lifestyle, improving medication management and helping to curb the appetite for alcohol may improve the chances of achieving abstinence.

Next, the patient must be taught to recognize the symptoms of both bipolar illness and cues to an impending relapse to drinking. Sometimes the two will overlap; sometimes they do not. Patients may simply not know when they are becoming ill. For such a patient, it would not be surprising if, rather than "people, places, and things" being relapse cues, the onset of a manic episode could be a signal that relapse is imminent. A change in sleep pattern, for example, going without sleep, or becoming preoccupied with an invention or grandiose schemes could be cues that the patient is likely to start drinking again. Explore with the patient what his or her pattern of using, cycles of mania and depression, and hospitalizations have been. This is not a patient whose behaviors will be modified in a season. But then, behaviors are not established over night. The more patients know about themselves, their illness, and relapses, the better the patient will be able to guard against succumbing to, or seeking help for, an increase in symptoms. In Chapter 16, there is an information checklist for patients. The intention is to educate patients to their illness and to help them learn to recognize changes in their moods. The patient then compares this checklist with changes in desire for, or actual use of, substances, in order to recognize personal patterns of use. Table 9-1 lists the issues addressed above.

CASE 9-1

Dan L., 23 years of age, is a man who has been smoking marijuana since the age of 15. Initially, he used it only on weekends with friends. After his first manic episode at the age of 17, the frequency of his use increased. He now smokes it daily and throughout the day. Because he is on probation for his second conviction for driving while intoxicated (DWI) he is concerned about the marijuana use. If his probation officer requests a random urine drug screen—and she will—his probation could be revoked and he could face jail time as a result. He has been abstinent of alcohol since his recent DWI, but has failed to curb

Table 9-1. Bipolar disorder: noncompliant patient

Issue	Effects and How Addressed
Revolving door patients	Frequent hospitalization Poor medication compliance Marginal functioning between hospitalizations Lack of structure
Patient motivation	Does the patient like or dislike hospitalizations, jail, and so on? Is the patient afraid he or she will be unable to change or afraid to try?

Medication choices	Mood stabilizers:
	    Lithium not a good choice with dual diagnosis
	    Valproic acid or carbamazepine better choices
	Antipsychotic
	    Typicals likely to increase substance use
	    Clozapine decreases use of substances
	Antidepressants
	    Tricyclic drugs increase incidence of rapid cycling
	    Most known about safety or efficacy of selective serotonin reuptake inhibitors

Alcohol use	Avoid disulfiram Naltrexone can be useful to counter craving Acamprosate may soon be available to counter craving
Patient knowledge	Increase knowledge regarding both conditions (see check list)

his marijuana smoking. When asked what marijuana does for him, the patient indicates it calms him down. In addition, he finds that the nausea and gastrointestinal discomfort that he has associated with his medication—valproic acid and carbamazepine—are relieved. The patient is working in a pizza restaurant. He smokes a joint shortly after rising in the morning. After he arrives at work, he smokes part of one while on break and part of one at noon. He does the same in the afternoon and as he is leaving to go home. Once home, he is not sure of how much he actually uses, but he admits he uses the entire evening until he goes to bed. The patient's psychiatric condition with his current medication, in the absence of alcohol, and in the presence of ongoing marijuana use, is stable. He has had no hospitalizations in more than 2 years. He appears to have difficulty learning and retaining new information and appears dull and unmotivated to make any improvement in his lifestyle, although he successfully completed 2 years of college with As and Bs. His family believes him to be capable of much higher functioning.

This patient is typical in several ways. First, it is more common for men with comorbid bipolar disorder and substance misuse to have had the latter briefly predate the overt signs of psychiatric symptoms. In addition, marijuana use did not occur in isolation, but rather concomitantly with alcohol use, and the latter has been the more problematic of the two. Finally, his heavy marijuana use, although not apparently worsening his psychosis, appears to be seriously sapping his motivation and perhaps keeping him from working up to his full potential.

It would be helpful to check both the valproate and carbamazepine levels. Some truth may exist to what the patient has to say about the gastrointestinal problem. Either of these agents can cause such side effects, each can alter the metabolism of the other, and the two can interfere with each other. Nausea and vomiting can occur with these agents, even at therapeutic levels, although they are more common at higher levels and cannabis is a well-known antinauseant and antiemetic. Of course, the possibility also exists that this is just rationalization too. Nevertheless, it is worth looking at it as a real possibility and to make dosage adjustments if the levels are in a toxic range. It appears that his mania has been controlled on this combination, thus, working with the existing medications should be a first effort.

It is often helpful, as Case 3-2 illustrated, to focus on how much of the patient's total income is dedicated to supporting his substance habit. This can be used as a jumping off point for attempting to establish goals. In the present case, the latter may be more complicated, however, because his ability to grasp and retain new information is being made more difficult by the presence of heavy cannabis use. On the other hand, he has one clear and well-established goal at the very beginning: he does not want to go to jail. Using that as one tangible goal, he could be helped to think of other rewards he will be able to afford as a result of saving his money and not buying more marijuana.

A major problem for this patient is his lack of structure in the evening. It appears that his job is helping limit his use during the daytime to some degree, but the lack of social support and un-structured nature of his evenings makes it possible for him to use large quantities of the drug during that time without any inter-ference. A couple of ways exist to address his daytime use. One, in regard to medication, will be addressed below. Another is to at-tempt to pair the patient with a "buddy" on breaks. This could be a family member, friend, coworker, or someone from a 12-step support group who could be relied on to be with the patient at break and lunch time, socialize with him, and distract him from using marijuana at those times.

If a dual disorders program exists for the patient in the evening so his job, which is providing income, insurance, and structure, will not be jeopardized, this would be an ideal situation. As few of these programs exist, another possibility would be attendance at a dual recovery support group, discussed in Chapter 2. Also, only a few of these are found. Thus, it may be necessary to work with the patient within the existing, although limited, structure. For example, if family is available, try to get them involved in the evening on a ro-tating basis to help provide support. Alternatively, the patient could be encouraged to volunteer in a nursing home, church, syna-gogue, or mosque; take a class; or engage in some activity where his presence is expected and his time structured.

Is there a need for a medication change? It is possible that the pa-tient only needed both mood stabilizers because of his heavy drink-ing. Which medication was used first? Was it ever effective alone? If so, for how long? Are there any clues why this changed? For ex-ample, did the patient's drinking or other substance use change at about the same time his response to medication changed?

If he never responded well to single agent treatment, another agent will need to be added as one medication is weaned. For ex-ample, if the history elicited is such that reason is seen to believe the patient will not do well on carbamazepine alone, gabapentin could be introduced while the valproate is reduced. Could the patient forego the midmorning marijuana at break and take gabapentin for its calming effect at that time instead? After a few days, could the afternoon break marijuana be dropped and another dose of gabapentin substituted?

Although this approach might take several weeks and frequent contact, it shows the patient that the clinician is listening to him, appreciates that discontinuing marijuana is uncomfortable, and that changing medication may help ease the process and meet some of the needs that marijuana previously supplied. Stopping the marijuana abruptly and completely would be the ideal, of course. Without structure and a social system to support ongoing abstinence, however, it is unlikely to succeed long term. Only by helping the patient to develop lifestyle changes and alternative behaviors is a lasting difference likely to be produced.

A special note should be made here about disulfiram in the con-text of marijuana use. As previously observed, a history of affective or psychotic disorders is a relative, not an absolute, contraindica-tion to disulfiram use. Ongoing marijuana use should be added as another caveat, as psychotic reactions have been reported to occur when disulfiram is added to marijuana, even in individuals with-out a history of preexisting psychosis (25,26). The issues addressed above are shown in Table 9-2.

Table 9-2.   Bipolar disorder: comorbid marijuana use

Issue	Effects and How Addressed
Marijuana use	Amotivational syndrome ?Use as an antiemetic
Medication issues	Possible toxicity: check blood levels Choice: both good medications: side effects described are possible Gabapentin and lamotrigine may be alternatives Changes should be gradual, with gradual weaning of one and introduction of other over time
Patient motivation	Focus on cost of use Focus on legal consequences, possibility of jail
Disulfiram use	Special issue here: reports of psychosis when cannabis and disulfiram combined, even in individuals without a history of psychosis
Social isolation	Use family, friends, employers, 12-Step members to assist patient in obtaining abstinence Involvement in dual recovery program, other activity beneficial Much time spent alone decreases likelihood of abstinence

CASE 9-2

Sarah B., a woman 28 years of age, has an 8-year history of crack cocaine use. She indicates that she began smoking crack shortly after the funeral of one of her sisters. A friend, commenting on her depression, told her the drug would help her mood, and indeed, it did. By the third occasion on which she used the drug, the patient found herself using in the same way her companions did (i.e., until her money or the cocaine ran out). For her, however, the cocaine did not seem to wear off. She continued to move too fast, to sleep not at all. Her sexual activity, heightened during her binge of cocaine, continued at an elevated and indiscriminate level, with multiple partners and without protection. She became loud and threatening to family members who seemed slow and ineffectual to her. Her family became frightened by her behavior and called police who thought her rapid speech and grandiosity required psychiatric care, not jail, and took her to the hospital. Since then, her pattern of behavior had been similar. The patient would take her medication as prescribed and refrain from cocaine use for several weeks at a time. Then, for no reason that she could identify, she would resume using the drug, and, after a few binges, end up in the hospital.

As noted, individuals with bipolar disorder often indicate that the allure of cocaine is that it induces a "high" (i.e., euphoria, heightened activity, energy, and sexual activity) just as mania does. Nothing special should be read into the fact that this patient began using cocaine during a period of depression. It could just as well have occurred during a period of mania. The issues are the same. Regrettably, only clozapine, a medication with many restrictions on its administration, has clearly been shown to decrease appetite for cocaine, although, as noted in Chapter 6, a number of agents have been tried.

It would be worthwhile to ask the patient specifically about the time interval between cocaine binges. Exactly what is "several weeks at a time?" Although she is unable to identify any reasons for her behavior, it is possible that the treatment provider can help her find one. A couple of obvious possibilities are a monthly cycle—one around the arrival of her disability check if she receives one, the other around her menstrual cycle. Premenstrual exacerbation of psychosis and depression are well-described phenomena, although the literature does not consistently support that it happens. If such does occur, it appears to be highly individual in nature. It is also suggested that women are more susceptible to substance use at this time (27–30).

If timeframe association is found, the patient should be encouraged to develop a strategy in advance for dealing with it. For example, she might see to it that she is not alone at all or has no transportation, money, or opportunity to buy any cocaine. She might arrange a trip somewhere that she knows no one will or will not be able to obtain her drug of choice. The idea is to be ready in advance and to have a plan in place before the anticipated time.

If no such clean relationship exists—and often it does not—it is still important to evaluate stresses and the individual's personal relapse cues to help her to develop a plan to avoid relapses in the future.

In terms of antidepressant treatment, the tricyclic desipramine has shown some benefit in decreasing cocaine use in a select population of depressed individuals. However, as emphasized, it appears that TCA greatly increase the risk of rapid cycling. Further, individuals with comorbid bipolar disorder and substance misuse, in general, and women, in particular, are already more susceptible to rapid cycling conditions. In addition, a risk exists of added cardiotoxicity and seizure activity when TCA and cocaine are combined. Thus, such cannot be recommended. Instead, an SSRI is the drug of choice, although unlikely to have a significant effect on cocaine craving.

It would be reasonable to ask the patient what her reason is for discontinuing her medications. Does she do this to become manic? Has she ever had a true depression other than the period of grieving described above? Is there something about her medications that she finds aversive? It is also necessary to assess the patient's baseline level of functioning. Is she ever truly euthymic or does she typically remain in only a partially treated hypomanic state?

If her motivation is to become manic, the treating clinician would do well to engage the patient and those around her in a discussion of the consequences of her actions. During manic episodes it is not uncommon for patients to lose friends, family, and money; engage in unsafe sexual activity; and break laws, resulting in incarceration or hospitalization. Has the cost of the brief pleasure been worth the time? If the answer is "yes" or the consequences have not yet been substantial, it may be helpful to enroll the patient in a mania support group where she can become acquainted with others who have not been so fortunate.

If the patient has ever had a true depression, it might be helpful to remind her that the condition of bipolar illness is unpredictable. Where she may be chasing the manic by discontinuing her medications, she may instead meet the depression. There is no guarantee of which mood she will experience. If she has not yet experienced mania's polar opposite, the clinician may only be able to point out that, statistically, it will happen, it will not be pleasant, and it can be life threatening.

Then is the issue of the medications themselves. Is there something about them that is objectionable? The vignette does not state precisely what medications the patient takes. At least, we can predict she is on a mood stabilizer. It has already been discussed at length that lithium is relatively ineffective in dually diagnosed individuals with bipolar disorder. What has not been discussed is that the approved mood stabilizers, lithium and valproic acid, are associated with substantial weight gain, as are most antipsychotic medications and many antidepressants. Patients quickly figure out that the many pounds they suddenly put on and cannot take off are a direct result of the prescriptions they are taking and resist taking them.

Although it is easy for the treatment provider to dismiss this as a trivial cosmetic issue compared with the problems the psychiatric condition causes if left untreated, it is not trivial to the individual who has to endure it. Not only does she have to accept the self-concept assault that she has a major mental illness, but the blow to the physical self-image as well. It is reasonable to probe about the issue.

If the patient admits this is part of the problem, the clinician can begin to work more closely around this issue. A first and obvious response is a dietitian consult. Many such patients admit to intense carbohydrate craving. Another problem is that the medications are sedating and patients simply become physically much less active, making it easier to gain and keep on the pounds. Encouraging increased activity or enrollment in an exercise program can serve both to help with the weight problem and to increase socialization.

Finally, manipulation of the medications may be in order. Increasing evidence indicates that topiramate may be associated with weight loss. Although this particular medication has not yet proved itself as a mood stabilizer, its use as an adjunct can help to counter the weight gain that antipsychotic and other medication use can cause.

This patient might also benefit from the worksheet introduced in Chapter 16, which asks patients to list what it is they want from their drug of choice, what they get from their drug of choice, and whether the two are the same. It further asks the patient to develop alternate strategies for obtaining these ends that are not

Table 9-3. **Bipolar disorder: comorbid cocaine use**

Issue	Effects and How Addressed
Cocaine use	Has patient suffered any consequences of use? Periodicity of use: is there a pattern? Arrival of disability check? Menstrual association? Desired result of use: to become manic? Currently no medications available to help counter craving
Weight gain	Can result from antipsychotic, antidepressant, mood stabilizer medication use May be motivation to stop medications Encourage increased exercise, dietary changes Use of topiramate may be beneficial
Medication	Avoid tricyclic antidepressants because of risk of inducing rapid cycling, increased seizure activity, and cardiotoxicity
Patient education	Educate patient to both illnesses, help develop alternate means of achieving result desired from using

likely to get the patient into trouble. Table 9-3 lists the issues addressed above.

REFERENCES

1. Haywood TW, Kravitz HM, Grossman LS, et al. Predicting the "revolving door": phenomenon among patients with schizophrenia, schizoaffective, and affective disorders. *Am J Psychiatry* 1995; 152(6):856–861.
2. Birmingham L. Between prison and the community: the 'revolving door psychiatric patient' of the nineties. *Br J Psychiatry* 1999; 174(5):378–379.
3. Shaner A, Eckman TA, Roberts LJ, et al. Disability income, cocaine use, and repeated hospitalization among schizophrenic cocaine abusers—a government sponsored revolving door? *N Engl J Med* 1995;333(12):777–783.
4. Pini S, Dell'Osso I, Mastrocinque C, et al. Axis I comorbity in bipolar disorder with psychotic features. *Br J Psychiatry* 1999;175: 467–471.
5. Nunes EV, McGrath PJ, Wager S, et al. Lithium treatment for cocaine abusers with bipolar spectrum disorders. *Am J Psychiatry* 1990;147(5):655–657.
6. Brady KT, Sonne SC, Anton R, et al. Valproate in the treatment of acute bipolar affective episodes complicated by substance abuse: a pilot study. *J Clin Psychiatry* 1995;56(3):118–121.
7. Sporn J, Sachs G. The anticonvulsant lamotrigine in treatment resistant manic depressive illness. *J Clin Psychopharmacol* 1997; 17(3):185–189.

8. Calabrese JR, Fatemi SH, Woyshville MJ. Antidepressant effects of lamotrigine in rapid cycling bipolar disorder. *Am J Psychiatry* 1996;153:1236.

9. Botts SR, Raskind J. Gabapentin and lamotrigine in bipolar disorder. *Am J Health Syst Pharm* 1999;56(19):1939–1944.

10. Zimmet SV, Strous RD, Burgess ES, et al. Effects of clozapine on substance use in patients with schizophrenia and schizoaffective disorder: a retrospective survey. *J Clinl Psychopharmacol* 2000; 20(1):94–98.

11. Hummel B, Dittmann S, Forsthoff A, et al. Clozapine as add-on medication in the maintenance treatment of bipolar and schizoaffective disorders: a case series. *Neuropsychobiology* 2002; 45(Suppl 1):37–42.

12. Brown ES, Thomas NR, Carmody T, et al. Atypical antipsychotics in bipolar and schizoaffective disorders. *Pharmacopsychiatry* 2001;34(2):80–81.

13. Guille C, Sachs GS, Ghaemi SN. A naturalistic comparison of clozapine, risperidone, and olanzapine in the treatment of bipolar disorder. *J Clin Psychiatry* 2000;61(9):638–642.

14. Ciapparelli A, Dell'Osso L, Pini S, et al. Clozapine for treatment refractory schizophrenia, schizoaffective disorder, and psychoactive bipolar disorder: a 24-month naturalistic study. *J Clin Psychiatry* 2000;61(5):329–334.

15. Buckley P, Thompson P, Way L, et al. Substance abuse among patients with treatment resistant schizophrenia: characteristics and implications for clozapine therapy. *Am J Psychiatry* 1994;151: 385–389.

16. Dunner DL. Rapid cycling bipolar affective disorders. In: Goldberg JF, Harrow M, eds. *Bipolar disorders: clinical course and outcome.* Washington, DC: American Psychiatric Press, 1999:199–218.

17. Volpicelli JR, Watson NT, King AC, et al. Effect of naltrexone on alcohol high in alcoholics. *Am J Psychiatry* 1995;152(4):613–615.

18. Volpicelli JR, Alterman AI, Hayashida M, et al. Naltrexone in the treatment of alcohol dependence. *Arch Gen Psychiatry* 1992;49: 876–880.

19. Sernyak MJ, Glazer WM, Heninger GR, et al. Naltrexone augmentation of neuroleptics in schizophrenia. *J Clin Psychopharmacol* 1998;18(3):248–251.

20. Marchesi GF, Santone G, Cotani P, et al. The therapeutic role of naltrexone in negative symptoms of schizophrenia. *Prog Neuropsychopharmacol Biol Psychiatry* 1995;19(8):1239–1249.

21. Welch EB, Thompson DF. Opiate antagonists for the treatment of schizophrenia. *J Clin Pharm Ther* 1994;19(5):279–283.

22. Kingsbury SJ, Salzman C. Disulfiram in the treatment of alcoholic patients with schizophrenia. *Hospital and Community Psychiatry* 1990;41(2):133–134.

23. Nunes E, Quitkin F. Disulfiram and bipolar affective disorder. *J Clin Psychopharmacol* 1987;7(4):284.

24. Bakish D, Lapierre YD. Disulfiram and bipolar affective disorder: a case report. *J Clin Psychopharmacol* 1986;6(3):178–180.

25. Mackie J, Clark D. Cannabis toxic psychosis while on disulfiram. *Br J Psychiatry* 1994;164(3):421.

26. Lacoursiere RB, Swatek R. Adverse interaction between disulfiram and marijuana: a case report. *Am J Psychiatry* 1983;140(2): 243–244.

27. Magharious W, Goff DC, Amico E. Relationship of gender and menstrual status to symptoms and medication side effects in patients with schizophrenia. *Psychiatry Res* 1998;77(3):159–166.
28. Harris AH. Menstrually related symptom changes in women with schizophrenia. *Schizophr Res* 1997;27(1):93–99.
29. Leibenluft E, Ashman SB, Feldman-Naim S, et al. Lack of relationship between menstrual cycle phase and mood in a sample of women with rapid cycling bipolar disorder. *Biol Psychiatry* 1999;46(4):577–580.
30. Hallonquist JD, Seeman MV, Lang M, et al. Variation in symptom severity over the menstrual cycle of schizophrenia. *Biol Psychiatry* 1993;33(3):207–209.

Major Depression and Substance Misuse

1. Demographics
   a. At any one time: 10%; lifetime: 17%
   b. Women twice as frequently as men
2. Medication issues
   a. Partial response rate: 90%
   b. High rate of relapse and recurrence even with maintenance medication
3. Problems caused by disorder
   a. Poorer overall functioning: poorer job performance, poorer physical health
   b. Increased risk of suicide
4. Etiology: may be a strong genetic component to development of a problem, with differential effect by gender
5. Comorbid substance misuse and depression common
   a. Comorbidity increases risk of suicide
   b. Nicotine
      i. Higher incidence of major depression among smokers
      ii. Presence of depression has prognostic significance in ability to stop smoking
   c. Alcohol
      i. Alcohol misuse makes diagnosing and treating depression difficult
      ii. Presence of depression has prognostic significance
   d. Cannabis
      i. Question of whether cannabis use is cause or result of depression
      ii. Data conflicting regarding effect of cannabis on depression
   e. Opioids
      i. Incidence of depression high in this population
      ii. Debate whether opioids act as a depressant or antidepressant
   f. Cocaine
      i. Suicidal behavior common
      ii. Premorbid depression may predispose to greater response to cocaine

BACKGROUND

Approximately 10% of the adult population suffers from major depression at any given time, according to studies both in the United States and in other countries, with up to 17% likely to suffer a depressive episode at some point in their lives (1–4). Women are twice as likely as men to suffer from depression (5). Whereas up to 90% of patients who receive antidepressant medication respond to treatment, a significant number fail to achieve full remission of symptoms (6). It is common for individuals with major depression to suffer both relapses to depression and recurrences of this mood disorder (7). Whereas relapse and recurrences can occur among individuals maintained on antidepressants, it is less likely than among those who discontinue pharmacotherapy (7).

Clearly, individuals with major depression, in general, are less functional than their unimpaired counterparts. They are less productive on the job, present with more absenteeism and poorer health, and have a poorer prognosis when medically ill. In addition, most individuals who commit suicide have substance misuse, major depression, or both (8).

Genes play a strong part in predisposition to major depression, but the genetic effect may influence the genders differently (9). Onset of depression tends to occur before the age of 30, with women having both earlier onset and more severe symptoms than do men (10,11). Interestingly, evidence suggests the age of onset of depression is decreasing at a time when the age of onset of alcohol and other drug use disorders is decreasing as well (12).

SUBSTANCE MISUSE AND DEPRESSION

More data are available regarding the co-occurrence of alcohol with major depression than with other substances of abuse. However, according to information from the National Institutes of Health ". . . comorbidity of a variety of drug use disorders and major depression is pervasive in the general [US] population . . ." (8) It is often difficult to diagnose depression with substance misuse and easy to attribute depressive symptoms to the substance use. Yet, evidence is that depression precedes the onset of the substance use in a significant percentage of cases (13,14). In addition, the importance of identifying and treating depression cannot be overstated. Comorbidity dramatically increases the likelihood of suicidal ideation, serious suicide attempt, and completed suicide (Table 10-1).

DEPRESSION AND NICOTINE

Over the last decade an increasing body of data relates to the relationship between nicotine and depression. Some studies have shown a higher incidence of major depression among nicotine-dependent individuals than among those who are not (15). Numerous anecdotal reports and formal studies exist regarding the onset of depression in individuals both with and without a history of such when they stop smoking tobacco (16–18). Premorbid depression can have prognostic significance in that the higher the degree of depression, the less likely the individual is to complete smoking cessation treatment (19). One study showed that in a smoking cessation program, both those who abstained and those who did not had a higher incidence of depression than did the population as a whole (20). Breslau et al. (15) found that individuals with any anxiety disorder or major depression who attempted to discontinue nicotine use had more severe withdrawal symptoms than those who did not have these

Table 10-1.   A comparison of depression and comorbid depression

	Depression	Depression + Substance Misuse
Demographics	Female: Male 2:1	Female ≅ Male[a]
Onset	< 30 years of age	No data
Risk	↑ Suicide	↑↑↑ Suicide

[a]Comparable, although not clearly equal.

disorders. Salin-Pascual et al. (21) suggested that nicotine it-self might have an antidepressant effect. They applied trans-dermal nicotine patches to nonsmokers with major depression and demonstrated a marked improvement in affect among their study subjects.

DEPRESSION AND ALCOHOL

No question, the presence of an alcohol use disorder seriously compromises the clinician's ability to assess for major depres-sion. At one time, it was considered appropriate to refuse to treat depression in an alcoholic until the individual had been abstinent for 6 months. Reasons for such an approach included the realistic concern about alcohol–medication interactions. Be-lief was that medication would be ineffectual in the context of heavy alcohol use and the desire was to accurately assess whether the affective disorder was primary or secondary to al-cohol use (i.e., whether the heavy alcohol consumption was a cause, or result, of the depression). A number of studies have demonstrated that alcohol dependence or abuse co-occurs with major depression at a rate considerably above that of the gen-eral population (22,23).

Even among alcohol-abusing individuals who do not demon-strate a depressive disorder on entering treatment, more than one fourth develop such within a few years (24). It appears that this is not simply a chance co-occurrence. Much information has accumulated suggesting a common genetic predisposition for both alcoholism and depression (25–28).

Whereas many individuals meet diagnostic criteria for major depression when they enter treatment for alcoholism, for most, the symptoms remit spontaneously within a few days of absti-nence (29). Depressive symptoms that continue beyond 2 or 3 weeks of abstinence have prognostic value, however. Studies show that individuals with continued depressive symptoms are more likely to relapse after treatment than are those who do not. Thus, it is important that both disorders be treated con-comitantly (30–32).

Alcohol contributes to more than a quarter of deaths by sui-cide (33). Depressed alcoholics show suicidal ideation two thirds of the time, compared with nonalcoholic depressed peo-ple (34). Further, the presence of depression and alcoholism greatly increases the risk of serious suicide attempt or comple-tion (35–37). Again, such data strongly support the use of medica-tion in the actively drinking alcohol-dependent individual with a dual diagnosis.

CASE 10-1

Mr. S. had always been a man of action. Throughout his work-ing career he had been one relied on to get the job done. When his son needed educational help, Mr. S. contacted educators all over the country to find the best resources for addressing the problem. When his daughter's marriage went sour, he hired the best divorce lawyers to protect her interests. When his family confronted him about his drinking 3 years before, he had checked himself into a treatment program and had not touched a drop since. Finding the leading experts to treat his wife's breast cancer, however, had proved beyond him, and he seemed completely unprepared, at 72 years of age, to be retired and a widower with time on his hands. He thought about drinking again. Reading—previously a passion—no longer held any interest. Once a master woodworker, he had not touched the hope chest he had promised his daughter. More and more he found himself feeling hopeless, useless, and worthless. He did not want to hurt his children and grand-children by killing himself, but he was tired of the pain he was experiencing. Mr. S began considering suicide. He needed a way to kill himself that would be lethal—being a vegetable and the pain that would cause was not acceptable. He had a gun and wasn't afraid to use it, but what if one of the grandchildren found him? When he started drinking again—quietly, alone, without the knowledge of his family—he did not think he could possibly get any lower.

DEPRESSION AND MARIJUANA

Information regarding how cannabis affects mood is contra-dictory. Part of the problem lies in what constitutes a "heavy" dose of δ-9 tetrahydrocannabinol (THC) and who is an "occa-sional" user of the drug. Some studies show that depression is more common among heavy users of THC, defined as daily users, when compared with occasional users (38,39). Some data show that the highest depression scores are found among the heavi-est users (40), suggesting a dose-dependent relationship be-tween depression and THC. It is further suggested that the so-called "amotivational syndrome" is actually depressive symp-toms in heavy smokers of cannabis (41). One large epidemiologic study looked at a population with a baseline history of mari-juana use but not depression. At 15-year followup, the mari-juana users were at a fourfold increased risk for depression and suicidal ideation when compared with those who, at baseline, had neither cannabis use nor depressive symptoms (42). The op-posite view is argued by one large multicenter study suggesting that THC use followed the onset of depression, lending support to the self-medication hypothesis. Finally, one set of researchers suggests that marijuana itself may act as an antidepressant in some populations (43).

DEPRESSION AND OPIOIDS

Data regarding opioid users must be viewed with caution, as much of the information available has been obtained from pa-tients in methadone maintenance programs and may not be re-flective of opioid users as a whole. In addition, opioid users tend to use other drugs as well, typically alcohol, cocaine, or benzo-diazepines (44–46). Nevertheless, it is known that opioid addicts tend to have a higher incidence of major depression compared with the general population, both in the United States and else-where (47–49). Although some researchers have suggested that the dysphoria encountered among opioid-dependent patients is a result of the drug's effects, it appears that premorbid depression also occurs in a substantial number of opioid addicts (50). Further, as is discussed below, observers have noted an increase in anger and depressive symptoms when opioids were removed, rather than the converse.

As in the case with other substances of abuse, depression can be safely and effectively treated with medication even in individuals who are actively using opioids (51–53). Also, as in the case of other substances, treating the depression may result in a reduction in opioid use, although this effect is not as pronounced as it is when alcohol consumption is reduced in patients with depression, for example.

It has long been recognized that opioids themselves have significant antidepressant properties, and use of these substances for this purpose was an accepted practice at one time. Dependence on this class of drugs, however, has made them less desirable for this purpose. New research using mixed agonist–antagonists, however, has focused on this class of drugs once again for the treatment of refractory depression (54,55).

DEPRESSION AND PSYCHOSTIMULANTS

Suicidal behavior is common among cocaine users. One landmark study found that one third of completed suicides in a 1-year period in the early 1990's were positive for cocaine or its metabolites (56,57). Some evidence suggests that individuals with premorbid major depression experience a more robust response to cocaine administration, further reinforcing their use of the drug (58,59). Where continued depressive symptoms predict relapse among those who misuse alcohol, studies have not consistently shown that cocaine users who continue to show depression are more likely to relapse to cocaine than do those who do not, although numbers are small (60–62).

MEDICATIONS AND SUBSTANCES OF ABUSE

Nicotine

Bupropion is the most widely accepted medication used as an aide to smoking cessation, but no studies have looked at whether it has a differential effect on smokers versus nonsmokers. In fact, most studies do not address this issue. One study suggests that fluoxetine might show some benefit in helping only those smokers who were depressed in establishing abstinence (63,64).

Alcohol

Imipramine, lithium, fluoxetine, and nefazodone are among the medications that have been directly studied for treating depression in actively drinking alcoholics (65–69). All have been successful to some degree in decreasing alcohol consumption and improving depressive symptoms. The risk of dehydration and concomitant lithium intoxication, with its attendant risks, limits its usefulness in actively drinking alcoholics, however. The additive effects of tricyclic antidepressants (TCA) (e.g., imipramine) when combined with alcohol, in addition to the high risk of suicide in depressed alcoholics, makes this combination less desirable without strict supervision and restriction of the amount of the drug available to the patient. Reports of hepatotoxicity associated with nefazodone have appeared recently (69a, 69b). Thus, more data are needed before this agent can be deemed safe in actively drinking alcoholics. Selective serotonin reuptake inhibitors (SSRI) do not appear to cause significant problems when taken by actively drinking alcoholics according to Ciraulo et al. (70) and may be the safest medications currently available for treating depressed alcoholics who continue to drink.

Psychostimulants

A number of medications have been tried with cocaine users, both depressed and not depressed, to decrease craving, improve retention in treatment, and treat depressive symptoms. To date, no evidence indicates that dopamine agonists or any antidepressant medications reduce craving or improve retention in treatment (62,71). In addition, a question exists whether TCA and cocaine, either of which can increase the likelihood of cardiotoxicity, could pose an additive risk to the patient. This is a theoretic risk, no reports have been found (70).

Marijuana

Little information is available regarding interaction between antidepressant medications and cannabis. Cornelius et al. (72) suggest that fluoxetine can help decrease both depressive symptoms and marijuana use in depressed marijuana users. One study looked at bupropion as an agent that perhaps might attenuate withdrawal symptoms with marijuana abstinence and found that it actually made the syndrome significantly worse (73). Another group reports four cases of adolescents on tricyclic medications for attention deficit disorder who showed delirium and cognitive changes after smoking marijuana (74).

Opioids

Tricyclic antidepressants and SSRI alike, as well as nefazodone, all appear to increase the analgesic effects of opioids. Sertraline has been found to cause an initial increase in methadone levels, when introduced, although this gradually returns to baseline without further adjustment of methadone dosage (75). Some evidence shows that simply stabilizing opioid addicts on methadone results in improvement in depressive symptoms with no additional benefit from fluoxetine (76). Anecdotal reports indicate that fluvoxamine may inhibit the metabolism of methadone, an effect that was exploited beneficially in one case and had near fatal consequences in another (77,78). It is too soon to tell if nefazodone, with its new hepatotoxicity warnings, will prove safe in this population, which has a high incidence of hepatitis B and C. TCA have been effectively used to treat depression in patients on methadone maintenance. It is also well known in methadone maintenance clinics, however, that patients buy and sell such agents as amitriptyline to exploit their sedative and anticholinergic properties. This makes SSRIs preferable medications to use. It is also known that this practice exists outside of methadone clinics as well (79) (Table 10-2).

Table 10-2.   Substance use and depression

Substance	Incidence of Use in Depression	Effect on Treatment	Medication Effects	Other Issues
Nicotine	Higher among smokers than nonsmokers	↑ Rate of dropout from treatment	↓ Levels of imipramine, amitryptiline, nortriptyline	Depression → ↑ withdrawal sxs nicotine cessation → ↑ depressive sxs even without premorbid history Antidepressant properties of its own?
Alcohol	↑ Incidence of depression among alcohol users and abusers	Continued depression with abstinence → ↑ likelihood of relapse	Lithium → dehydration TCAs: → additive effect Selective serotonin reuptake inhibitors: no known problem	↑ Risk of suicide Common genetic predisposition to alcohol and depression?

Major Depression and Substance Misuse 125

Cannabis	? Presence of depression dose related (i.e., effect of cannabis?)	Data contradictory: cause or consequence?	Bupropion → worsen withdrawal ? Delirium with TCA	
Opioids	↑ Incidence of depression	Stabilization on methadone associated with ↓ in depressive sxs	No benefit of fluoxetine Transient ↑ in methadone levels with sertraline Fluvoxamine inhibits metabolism	? Antidepressant effect of methadone and other opioids
Psychostimulants	Premorbid depression →stronger response to cocaine (↑ reinforcing effect)	Increased depression → ↑ risk of relapse	Theoretic: TCA + cocaine ↑ cardiotoxicity	

sxs, symptoms; TCA, tricyclic antidepressant.

REFERENCES

1. Spaner D, Bland RC, Newman SC. Epidemiology of psychiatric disorders in Edmonton. Major depressive disorder. *Acta Psychiatr Scand* 1994;Suppl 376:7–15.
2. Fichter MM, Narrow W, Roper M, et al. Sociodemographic factors and prevalence rates of mental illness in Germany and the United States. *J Nerv Ment Dis* 1997;185(4):276–277.
3. Strock M. *Plain talk about depression.* Bethesda, MD: National Institute of Mental Health, 2000:1–25.
4. Kringlen E, Torgersen S, Cramer V. A Norwegian psychiatric epidemiological study. *Am J Psychiatry* 2001;158(7):1091–1098.
5. Kaplan HI, Sadock BJ. *Synopsis of psychiatry: behavioral sciences / clinical psychiatry.* Baltimore, MD: Lippincott Williams & Wilkins, 1998.
6. Mueller TI, Leon AC. Recovery, chronicity, and levels of psychopathology in major depression. In: Keller MB, ed. *Psychiatric Clin North Am,* Vol. 19. Philadelphia: WB Saunders, 1996;19:85–103.
7. Nierenberg AA, Alpert JE. Depressive breakthrough. In: Nierenberg AA, ed. *Depression: recent developments and innovative treatments,* Vol 23. Philadelphia: WB Saunders, 2000:731–742.
8. NIMH. *In harm's way: suicide in America.* Rockville, MD: National Institute of Mental Health, 2001.
9. Kendler KS, Prescott CA. A population based twin study of lifetime major depression in men and women. *Arch Gen Psychiatry* 1999;56(1):39–44.
10. Daley SE, Hammen C, Rao U. Predictors of first onset and recurrence of major depression in young women during the five years following high school graduation. *J Abnorm Psychol* 2000;109(3):525–533.
11. Kornstein SG, Schatzberg AF, Thase ME, et al. Gender differences in chronic major and double depression. *J Affect Disord* 2000;60(1):1–11.
12. Burke KC, Burke JDJ, Rae DS, et al. Comparing age of onset of major depression and other psychiatric disorders by birth cohorts in five US community populations. *Arch Gen Psychiatry* 1991;48(9):789–795.
13. Grant BF, Harford TC. Comorbidity between DSM-IV alcohol use disorders and major depression: results of a national survey. *Drug Alcohol Depend* 1995;39(3):197–206.
14. Abraham HD, Fava M. Order of onset of substance abuse and depression in a sample of depressed outpatients. *Compr Psychiatry* 1999;40(1):44–50.
15. Breslau N, Kilbey MM, Andreski P. Nicotine dependence, major depression, and anxiety in young adults. *Arch Gen Psychiatry* 1991;48(12):1069–1074.
16. Bock BC, Goldstein MG, Marcus BH. Depression following smoking cessation in women. *J Subst Abuse* 1996;8(1):137–144.
17. Niaura R, Britt DM, Borrelli B, et al. History and symptoms of depression among smokers during a self initiated quit attempt. *Nicotine Tob Res* 1999;1(3):251–157.
18. Stage KB, Glassman AH, Covey LS. Depression after smoking cessation: case reports. *J Clin Psychiatry* 1996;57(10):467–469.
19. Curtin L, Brown RA, Sales SD. Determinants of attrition from cessation treatment in smokers with a history of major depressive disorder. *Psychol Addict Behav* 2000;14(2):134–142.

20. Tsoh JY, Humfleet GL, Munoz RF, et al. Development of major depression after treatment for smoking cessation. *Am J Psychiatry* 2000;157(3):368–374.

21. Salin-Pascual RJ, Rosas M, Jimenez-Genchi A, et al. Antidepressant effect of transdermal nicotine patches in nonsmoking patients with major depression. *J Clin Psychiatry* 1996;57(9): 387–389.

22. Grant BF, Harford TC, Dawson DA. Prevalence of DSM-IV alcohol abuse and dependence: United States, 1992. *Alcohol Health and Research World* 1994;18(3):243–248.

23. Regier DA, Farmer ME, Rae DS, et al. Comorbidity of mental disorders with alcohol and other drug abuse: results from the Epidemiological Catchment Area study. *JAMA* 1990;264(19): 2511–2518.

24. Coryell W, Endicott J, Keller M. Major depression in a nonclinical sample. *Arch Gen Psychiatry* 1992;49:117–125.

25. Nurnberger JIJ, Foroud T, Flury L, et al. Evidence for a locus on chromosome 1 that influences vulnerability to alcoholism and affective disorder. *Am J Psychiatry* 2001;158(5):718–724.

26. Gilman SE, Abraham HD. A longitudinal study of the order of onset of alcohol dependence and major depression. *Drug Alcohol Depend* 2001;63(3):277–286.

27. Kasperowicz-Dabrowiecka A, Rybakowski JK. Beyond the Winokur concept of depression spectrum disease: which types of alcoholism are related to primary affective illness? *J Affect Disord* 2001; 63(1–3):133–138.

28. Prescott CA, Aggen SH, Kendler KS. Sex specific genetic influences on the comorbidity of alcoholism and major depression in a population based sample of US twins. *Arch Gen Psychiatry* 2000; 57(8):803–811.

29. Schuckit MAT, Jayson E, Bergman M. Comparison of induced and independent major depressive disorders in 2945 alcoholics. *Am J Psychiatry* 1997;154:948–957.

30. Brower KJ, Aldrich MS, Robinson EA, et al. Insomnia, self-medication, and relapse to alcoholism. *Am J Psychiatry* 2001; 158(3):399–404.

31. Curran GM, Glynn HA, Kirchner J, et al. Depression after alcohol treatment as a risk factor for relapse among male veterans. *J Subst Abuse Treat* 2000;19(3):259–265.

32. Driessen M, Meier S, Hill A, et al. The course of anxiety, depression and drinking behaviors after completed detoxification in alcoholics with and without comorbid anxiety and depressive disorders. *Alcohol Alcohol* 2001;36(3):249–255.

33. Murphy GE, Wetzel RD, Robins E, McEvoy L. Multiple risk factors predict suicide in alcoholism. *Arch Gen Psychiatry* 1992;49: 459–463.

34. Cornelius JR, Salloum IM, Mezzich J, et al. Disproportionate suicidality in patients with comorbid major depression and alcoholism. Am J Psychiatry 1995;152(3):358–364.

35. Blair-West GW, Cantor CH, Mellsop GW, et al. Lifetime suicide risk in major depression: sex and age determinants. *J Affect Disord* 1999;55(2–3):171–178.

36. Petronis KR, Samuels JF, Moscicki EK, et al. An epidemiologic investigation of potential risk factors for suicide attempts. *Soc Psychiatry Psychiatr Epidemiol* 1990;25(4):193–199.

37. Salloum IM, Mezzich JE, Cornelius J, et al. Clinical profile of comorbid major depression and alcohol use disorders in an initial psychiatric evaluation. *Compr Psychiatry* 1995;36(4):260–266.
38. Degenhardt L, Hall W, Lynskey M. The relationship between cannabis use, depression and anxiety among Australian adults: findings from the National Survey of Mental Health and Well Being. *Soc Psychiatry Psychiatr Epidemiol* 2001;36(5):219–227.
39. Green BE, Ritter C. Marijuana use and depression. *J Health Soc Behav* 2000;41(1):40–49.
40. Troisi A, Pasini A, Saracco M, et al. Psychiatric symptoms in male cannabis users not using other illicit drugs. *Addiction* 1998;93(4):487–492.
41. Musty RE, Kaback L. Relationships between motivation and depression in chronic marijuana users. *Life Sci* 1995;56(23–24):2151–2158.
42. Bovasso GB. Cannabis abuse as a risk factor for depressive symptoms. *Am J Psychiatry* 2001;158(12):2033–2037.
43. Gruber AJ, Pope HGJ, Brown ME. Do patients use marijuana as an antidepressant? *Depression* 1996;4(2):77–80.
44. Weiss RD, Martinez-Raga J, Hufford C. The significance of a co-existing opioid use disorder in cocaine dependence: an empirical study. *Am J Drug Alcohol Abuse* 1996;22(2):173–184.
45. Kidorf M, Brooner RK, King VL, et al. Concurrent validity of cocaine and sedative dependence diagnoses in opioid-dependent outpatients. *Drug Alcohol Depend* 1996;42(2):117–123.
46. Ross J, Darke S. The nature of benzodiazepine dependence among heroin users in Sydney, Australia. *Addiction* 2000;95(12):1785–1793.
47. Brooner RK, King VL, Kidorf M, et al. Psychiatric and substance use comorbidity among treatment seeking opioid abusers. *Arch Gen Psychiatry* 1997;54(1):71–80.
48. Torrens M, San L, Peri JM, et al. Cocaine abuse among heroin addicts in Spain. *Drug Alcohol Depend* 1991;27(1):29–34.
49. Hendriks VM, Steer RA, Platt JJ, et al. Psychopathology in Dutch and American heroin addicts. *International Journal of the Addictions* 1990;25(9):1051–1053.
50. Handelsman L, Aronson MJ, Ness R, et al. The dysphoria of heroin addiction. *Am J Drug Alcohol Abuse* 1992;18(3):275–287.
51. Nunes EV, Quitkin FM, Donovan SJ, et al. Imipramine treatment of opiate-dependent patients with depressive disorders: a placebo-controlled trial. *Arch Gen Psychiatry* 1998;55(2):153–160.
52. Titievsky J, Seco G, Barranco M, et al. Doxepin as adjunctive therapy for depressed methadone maintenance patients: a double blind study. *J Clin Psychiatry* 1982;43(11):454–456.
53. Woody GE, O'Brien CP, Rickels K. Depression and anxiety in heroin addicts: a placebo-controlled study of doxepin in combination with methadone. *Am J Psychiatry* 1975;132(4):447–450.
54. Bodkin JA, Zornberg GL, Lukas SE, et al. Buprenorphine treatment of refractory depression. *J Clin Psychopharmacol* 1995;15(1):49–57.
55. Gold MS, Pottash AC, Sweeney D, Martin D, et al. Antimanic, antidepressant, and antipanic effects of opiates: clinical, neuro-anatomical, and biochemical evidence. *Ann NY Acad Sci* 1982;398:140–150.

56. Marzuk PM, Tardiff K, Leon AC, et al. Prevalence of cocaine use among residents of New York City who committed suicide during a one-year period. *Am J Psychiatry* 1992;149(3):371–375.

57. Roy A. Characteristics of cocaine dependent patients who attempt suicide. *Am J Psychiatry* 2001;158(8):1215–1219.

58. Sofuoglu M, Brown S, Babb DA, et al. Depressive symptoms modulate the subjective and physiological response to cocaine in humans. *Drug Alcohol Depend* 2001;63(2):131–137.

59. Kelder SH, Murray NG, Orpinas P, et al. Depression and substance use in minority middle school students. *Am J Public Health* 2001;91(5):761–766.

60. Bobo JK, McIlvain HE, Leed-Kelly A. Depression screening scores during residential drug treatment and risk of drug use after discharge. *Psychiatr Serv* 1998;49(5):693–695.

61. Brown RA, Monti PM, Myers MG, et al. Depression among cocaine abusers in treatment: relation to cocaine and alcohol use and treatment outcome. *Am J Psychiatry* 1998;155(2):220–225.

62. Schmitz JM, Stotts AL, Averill PM, et al. Cocaine dependence with and without comorbid depression: a comparison of patient characteristics. *Drug Alcohol Depend* 2000;60(2):189–198.

63. Hitsman B, Spring B, Borrelli B, et al. Influence of antidepressant pharmacotherapy on behavioral treatment adherence and smoking cessation outcome in a combined treatment involving fluoxetine. *Exp Clin Psychopharmacol* 2001;9(4):355–362.

64. Hitsman B, Pingitore R, Spring B, et al. Antidepressant pharmacotherapy helps some cigarette smokers more than others. *J Consult Clin Psychol* 1999;67(4):547–554.

65. McGrath PJ, Nunes EV, Stewart JW, et al. Imipramine treatment of alcoholics with primary depression: a placebo controlled clinical trial. *Arch Gen Psychiatry* 1996;535(3):232–240.

66. Cornelius JR, Sallou IM, Ehler JG, et al. Fluoxetine in depressed alcoholics: a double-blind, placebo-controlled trial. *Arch Gen Psychiatry* 1997;54(8):700–705.

67. Roy-Byrne PP, Pages KP, Russo JE, et al. Nefazodone treatment of major depression in alcohol-dependent patients: a double blind placebo controlled trial. *J Clin Psychopharmacol* 2000; 20(2):129–136.

68. Young LD, Patel M, Keeler MH. The effect of lithium carbonate on alcoholism in 20 male patients with concurrent major affective disorder. *Currents in Alcoholism* 1981;8:175–181.

69. Pond SM, Becker CE, Vandervoort R, et al. An evaluation of the effects of lithium in the treatment of chronic alcoholism I: clinical results. *Alcohol Clin Exp Res* 1981;5(2):247–251.

69a. Aranda-Michel J, Koehler A, Beharano P, et al. Nefazodone-induced liver failure: report of three cases. *Ann Intern Med* 1999; 130(4):285–288.

69b. Schirren CA, Baretton G. Nefazodone-induced acute liver failure. *Am J Gastroenterol* 2000; 95(6):1596–1597.

70. Ciraulo DA, Creelman WL, Shader RI, et al. Cyclic antidepressants. In: Ciraulo DA, Shader RI, Greenblatt, et al., eds. *Drug interactions in psychiatry*. Baltimore, MD: Williams & Wilkins, 1995:430.

71. Batki SL, Washburn AM, Delucchi K, et al. A controlled trial of fluoxetine in crack cocaine dependence. *Drug Alcohol Depend* 1996;41(2):137–142.

72. Cornelius JR, Salloum IM, Haskett RF, et al. Fluoxetine versus placebo for the marijuana use of depressed alcoholics. *Addict Behav* 1999;24(1):111–114.

73. Haney M, Ward AS, Comer SD, et al. Bupropion SR worsens mood during marijuana withdrawal in humans. *Psychopharmacology* 2001;155(2):171–179.

74. Wilens TE, Biederman J, Spender TJ. Case study: adverse effects of smoking marijuana while receiving tricyclic antidepressants. *J Am Acad Child Adolesc Psychiatry* 1997;36(1):45–48.

75. Hamilton SP, Nunes EV, Janal M, et al. The effect of sertraline on methadone plasma levels in methadone maintenance patients. *Am J Addict* 2000;9(1):63–69.

76. Petrakis I, Carroll KM, Nich C, et al. Fluoxetine treatment of depressive disorders in methadone maintained opioid addicts. *Drug Alcohol Depend* 1998;50(3):221–226.

77. DeMaria PA, Serota RD. A therapeutic use of the methadone fluvoxamine drug interaction. *J Addict Dis* 1999;18(4):5–12.

78. Alderman CP, Frith PA. Fluvoxamine-methadone interaction. *Aust N Z J Psychiatry* 1999;33(1):99–101.

79. Delisle JD. A case of amitriptyline abuse. *Am J Psychiatry* 1990; 147(10):1377–1378.

Treatment of Depression and Substance Misuse

1. Patient at high risk for suicide
   a. Risk factors reviewed
   b. Patient's age increases risk of injury caused by drinking alcohol
   c. Typical diagnostic tools may not be applicable in working with older adults
   d. Increased age a relative contraindication for outpatient detoxification
   e. Need for and choices of antidepressants
2. Patient with alcohol abuse and sleep disturbance
   a. Issues regarding effect of alcohol on sleep
   b. Options for increasing patient's social contacts and decreasing isolation
   c. Options for medication presented and similar to above
3. Cannabis and depression
   a. Issues regarding impact of cannabis level on mood and cognition
   b. Discussion of whether to treat symptoms of marijuana abstinence and choice of medications
4. Cocaine and depression
   a. Cocaine use carries substantial physical and psychiatric risks and patient presented is at high risk of both
   b. The period of depression following cocaine use should be over within 2 or 3 days, but carries with it a serious risk of suicide during that time
   c. Patient requires an environment that is conducive to remaining drug free
   d. Pros and cons of various antidepressant medications
5. Depression and opiates
   a. A pain patient with depression and iatrogenic dependence on opiates
   b. Opiates themselves may have antidepressant qualities: a patient attempting to decrease opiate use becomes suicidal
   c. Interactive effect of tricyclic antidepressant medications and opiates and how to exploit this effect
   d. Various methods of detoxifying an older individual with multiple medical problems

INTRODUCTION

Consider, patient Mr. S. (see Case 10-1): Does he need to be detoxified from alcohol? We know nothing about this patient's drinking pattern or the quantity he is drinking, so it is not possible to answer the question at this juncture. No question, he is severely depressed. More worrisome still, he has a number of the factors that place him in the highest risk category for suicide: older, male, history of alcohol misuse, and recent significant personal loss. His safety must be constantly kept in mind as a primary concern. Mr. S. is a patient at very high risk.

In addition, this patient presents the clinician with further challenges simply as a result of his age. Being an older adult, alcohol will affect him differently now than it did when he was younger. Because of changes in the volume of distribution that occurs with increasing age, his body does not tolerate the same amount of alcohol it did when he was younger. His bones are more fragile and he is more susceptible to falls and fractures. His cognition will be suffering more as a result as well.

Further, Mr. S. is a patient who, were it not that he is a self-professed alcoholic who has been in recovery, would normally not be diagnosed by his physician as having a drinking problem. The medical establishment is notoriously poor at diagnosing alcoholism in older middle class patients. Physicians fail to inquire about such things.

When they do, accepted screening tools (e.g., the CAGE [cut down, annoyed by criticism, guilty about drinking, eye-opener drinks] questionnaire) are unreliable in the geriatric population (1,2). Thus, under most conditions, a patient at such high risk as Mr. S. would not have his condition diagnosed and, hence, not be treated.

In general, as with younger individuals with comorbid alcohol problems and depression, the elderly can benefit from concomitant treatment of depression and substance misuse (3,4). If Mr. S. is drinking every day and throughout the day, however, no antidepressant will be of substantial benefit. Regardless of his drinking patterns, his age and his isolation dictate that hospitalization, at the very least for stabilization and observation, is indicated. He is not a candidate for outpatient detoxification. It is also likely that an inpatient psychiatric stay—involuntarily if necessary—is going to be required to ensure his safety. He is covertly drinking and it may not be possible to trust his promise to apprise others if he becomes more convinced that suicide is his only way out. His family needs to be heavily involved in his treatment. As has already been pointed out, this is a gentleman in the highest risk category for suicide and his risk of self-harm cannot be overstated.

Studies show that a wide variety of antidepressants can be effective, even in the face of actively drinking alcohol abusers, as discussed in Chapter 10. However, lack of safety makes it inadvisable to use agents such as monoamine oxidase inhibitors or tricyclic antidepressants (TCA) in patients who are abusing alcohol (5,6). Further, alcohol appears to increase the turnover rate of TCA, thus reducing the level and efficacy of these medications (7). Bupropion is well known to lower the seizure threshold and, thus, would be a medication to monitor closely if administered to an actively drinking alcoholic, and then only if he had no history of seizures.

Venlafaxine's extensive hepatic metabolism makes it a less desirable medication to treat the actively drinking alcohol user with any degree of liver dysfunction. Lack of experience using mirtazapine in this population makes it too early to know whether this will be a good treatment for this population. Serotonin reuptake inhibitors (SSRI) are effective in decreasing depressive symptoms in alcoholic patients without causing significant negative interactions (8). Mr. S. should be placed on an SSRI of the clinician's choosing and titrated to a dose that proves effective (Table 11-1).

CASE 11-1

Ms. L., 38 years of age, has a sleep problem. Over the last 6 years, since the birth of her third and last child, she has had increasing difficulty getting to and staying asleep. Initially, she was afraid to go to sleep for fear she would fail to hear her infant if he cried. Her second infant had died at 6 weeks of age of sudden infant death syndrome (SIDS). She harbored the suspicion

*that if she had heard the baby cry, she might have saved her life.
When she finally began to relax a bit at night when her third child
was about 3 years of age, she found she was unable to fall asleep
without first having a glass or two of wine or whiskey. Once
asleep, she discovered it was impossible to remain so. Instead, she
would waken at 2 or 3 AM and be unable to return to sleep. She
tossed and turned, replaying events of the day. Ms. L. often casti-
gated herself for shortcomings, both real and imagined, and found
herself worrying about things over which she could not possibly
exert any control. Ms. L. dragged through the days with no energy.
She felt trapped in her job and in her life, and had no hope for her
future. It sometimes seemed as though all she did was cry. Ms. L.
sometimes thought about suicide, but knew she could not take that
way out. Her husband had left them after the youngest was born,
and she had responsibilities to the children. Still, although she
loved them, she had no patience and was short tempered with her
two surviving sons. The only enjoyment she found was the increasing amount of alcohol she consumed at night.*

As always in dealing with alcohol, ask the question of whether
the patient requires help with detoxification. If Ms. L. is not mis-
representing her usage pattern, that is she drinks only at night
and is able to function throughout the day without any alcohol,
she is unlikely to need help with withdrawal. However, as she ob-
serves, she is going to suffer from significant sleep difficulties.
Ms. L. describes a common scenario, presenting with the com-
plaint that she is unable to sleep without a drink or two. Patients
often present in this fashion. They may recognize that the "one or
two" is becoming half a pint or a pint; on the rare occasion they do
skip a night, however, they are truly unable to sleep. Patients, and

Table 11-1.   Risk for suicide (Mr. S.) (see Case 10-1)

Issue	Effects and How Addressed
Risks of alcohol use because of age	Changes in volume of distribution of alcohol Changes in body's acceptance of alcohol Increased risk of cognitive or physical damage as a result of alcohol use Appropriate setting for detoxification if indicated: not a candidate for outpatient detox
Ongoing depression	Meets criteria for highest suicide risk Patient safety a constant concern Choice of appropriate medication important
Unresolved grief or isolation	Recent loss of spouse or recent retirement Family involvement beneficial Social isolation or withdrawal important factors Lack of structure needs to be addressed

even some clinicians, look at alcohol as a sleep aide, and in fact, it does help induce sleep. The sleep it promotes, however, is far from restful, as it suppresses rapid eye movement (REM) sleep, which is necessary for sleep to be replenishing (9). Thus, when Ms. L. awakens she does not feel refreshed. In addition, when the alcohol abuser tries to abstain, the sleep disturbance worsens. The individual will then be unable to get to sleep or stay asleep, often for many weeks. Although this will right itself eventually, it can last longer than the patient is able or willing to tolerate. Ms. L. is very vulnerable at this stage. As noted in the previous chapter, ongoing depression and sleep disturbance can be relapse cues to the individual in early recovery.

It may be best to help the patient by giving her something to help her sleep and, thus, engage her in the recovery process, rather than making her feel rejected or that no one is listening by saying "it will get better." Whereas an enormous variety of possible sleep-inducing drugs could be given, it is always useful to try to identify the source of the problem. Barring a primary sleep disorder, a problem well beyond the scope of this book, depression, anxiety, and alcohol are the most likely contributors here. Clearly, Ms. L. meets the criteria for major depression. Although the alcohol itself is likely worsening the problem at this point, dealing with the patient's depression may address the sleep issue as well.

In addition, Ms. L. must be helped to find some activity to substitute for her substance-using behavior, ideally at the same time when she is at the highest risk for using. Attending a 12-step meeting could be a substitute, for example, although other possibilities exist as well. Finding something for Ms. L. may be difficult. She is an isolative drinker—alone at night when the children are asleep. Thus, although attendance at a meeting could still be helpful, it is unlikely—unless she has a friend who can stay with the children while she goes out—that she can do so at the times that are hardest for her—in the lonely hours of the evening.

Perhaps Ms. L. could establish a rotating list of friends, family, 12-step members, or others willing to assist by calling at this high-risk time to give her moral support and encouragement while she is establishing her sobriety. In addition, encouraging her to join a support group for parents who have lost children to SIDS to help her deal with her grief and guilt may also be of benefit.

The same line of reasoning then applies with both Ms. L. and Mr. S. in terms of medication choices. It should be noted, however, that paroxetine is more sedating than other members of this drug family. It could serve the dual benefit of concomitantly improving her sleep and depression in this situation (Table 11-2).

CASE 11-2

Joe T., 25 years old, started having trouble in his teens. He wasn't sure where his father was half the time, but he was glad he wasn't around. It was quieter, since the fighting was only between him and his mother then. He went to school every day because his mother woke him up for it. She did not want him around. Joe T. would have his first joint on the way to school, a second and third during the day, and he wasn't sure how much later, as he was too wasted to count. He did not get into trouble

*with the law after he started smoking dope so heavily. Before, he
was angry and fighting all the time. He wanted to hurt people
and did not care if they hurt him. It felt good just to hit something or somebody. When he took up smoking "weed," he was
content to go to school, sit in class, and just watch the world
go by. In his twenties, his marijuana use declined, but did not
stop. He no longer spent the entire day stoned, but if he went
more than a day without using, he became irritable and hostile
and had difficulty concentrating. He also had trouble sleeping
and generally did not feel well. At this point, Joe knew he had
to give it up entirely and really wanted to do so. The cost bothered him. His new circle of friends did not get high with him.
And besides, he wanted to get a better job. Without being able
to pass a urine toxicology screen, he would not be able to get
any of the union jobs for which he was eligible. It was time to
get beyond this.*

In Chapter 10, it was pointed out that the relationship between depression and marijuana is difficult to untangle: cause
and effect are unclear. Most practitioners would recognize in the
early Joe T. the symptoms of adolescent male depression. Rather
than sitting in a corner crying, he acted out in a hostile and aggressive fashion that marijuana suppressed, rendering him apa-
thetic and much less aggressively angry. The irritability he
experiences now when he does not use cannabis could be symptomatic of the marijuana abstinence syndrome or of continued or
renewed depression.

It is often difficult to establish with any certainly that a given
patient has a premorbid history of depression. On the other hand,

Table 11-2. Alcohol abuse and sleep disturbance (case 11-1)

Issue	Effects and How Addressed
Sleep disturbance	Noted as a common relapse cue. In this case, likely a consequence of patient's depression
	Alcohol use further contributes to fatigue because of suppression of rapid eye movement sleep
Grief	Loss of a child, a severe stressor: patient in need of survivor support
Depression in addition to grief	Choice of medication important: similar line of reasoning as in previous case
Alcohol misuse and risk of relapse	Needs behavioral changes: involvement of family and friends. Network therapy may be of benefit if atten- dance at a 12-step or other support groups not possible

with Joe T., it is fairly clear. What is not so clear is what is happening right now.

It might help Joe T. to know how long he can expect to feel as he does if marijuana is the only problem. In some facilities, it is possible to obtain a δ-9 tetrahydrocannabinol (THC) level. Many laboratories obtain a screen only for drugs of abuse (i.e., a result that says the drug is or is not present). A drug level quantifies how much drug is present in the individual's body. This information can give the clinician a general idea of how much drug the patient has been using and how long it will take for the drug to leave his body. For example 50ηgm/dL is a low level, just detectable in many laboratories. Such a level would be unlikely to account for his symptoms. In addition, his screen will likely be negative in just a few days. A level of 350 ηg/dL, however, implies a high level of daily or several times a day usage and will likely take several weeks to become negative. Such a level could well be sufficient to account for the irritability being described. If obtaining a drug level is not possible, weekly drug screens might also be helpful. If he is not using cannabis but his toxicology screen remains positive for 4 or 5 weeks, it says his starting level was quite high.

While giving Joe T. some feedback to what he can expect in terms of symptoms and how long he can expect them to last, it is also important to determine if Joe T. is experiencing any other symptoms of depression. Most important, of course, are questions about safety and suicidal thoughts and plans. If he is safe and his THC level is high, it may be reasonable to treat him symptomatically and postpone antidepressant therapy for 1 or 2 weeks.

Some clinicians would argue that a patient such as Joe T. should not be medicated at all; he should be sent to 12-step meetings or to a treatment program and told to wait out the symptoms he is experiencing. It is true that the symptoms will improve without any treatment. However, a problem with this approach is the extremely high dropout rate associated with it. It would be easy to blame the dropout on the patient and say he simply was not motivated. However, it should be pointed out that many patients such as Joe T., at this stage, do not have the coping skills necessary to wait a month or more to feel comfortable and be able to rest. That is why they are asking for help. Their coping skill has always been their drug. Helping the patient now may not give the message that "every time something goes wrong, you take a pill." Rather, medication for symptomatic relief, instead, may give the message that "when you need and ask for help and support, brief, temporary medication intervention under clinical guidance may be permissible."

It would be reasonable to involve Joe T. in the decision-making process. What are the symptoms that are most troublesome to him? Sleep is likely to be one issue. For this, he would probably do as well with an over-the-counter medication than with anything the clinician would reasonably prescribe. Some excellent nonbenzodiazepine, nonbarbiturate sleeping agents are available to the clinician as well, should the prescriber have a preference.

Treatment of the irritability with nonaddicting agents is another service the treatment provider can offer. A large variety of

Table 11-3.   Cocaine use and depression (case 11-3)

Issues	Effects and How Addressed
Environment	Minimize contact with cocaine environment Association with nonusing friends Institutionalization if necessary
Depression	Suicide risk an issue regardless of whether depression is primary or secondary Secondary to cocaine: over within a few days Primary: treatment necessary
Medication choices	Theoretic risk of lowering seizure threshold No medication proved to decrease craving

medications have been used over the years for treatment of such symptoms, which are similar in many ways to nicotine cessation. This similarity is what prompted researchers to try bupropion with its well-recognized success in treating tobacco addiction. As noted, however, this was not at all successful (10).

Because of similarity to symptoms of nicotine withdrawal and the success clonidine has demonstrated in relieving some of these effects, it is one agent that has shown some success in relieving cannabis "withdrawal symptoms" (11–13). Joe T. could be begun on a clonidine patch and would likely notice some improvement in his irritability, lability, and general discomfort. Another agent that might be of benefit is trazodone (25 mg) twice daily and (50–100 mg) at bedtime for sleep. Whereas amitriptyline and some of its relatives have been used successfully for relief of symptoms such as Joe T. has, some reported problems with delirium and the abuse of tricyclics by this and opiate-abusing populations make this a less advisable alternative.

CASE 11-3

Ms. D. recalls few times in her life when she didn't feel depressed. It was a surprise to her to find out that not everyone thinks about suicide or sometimes wishes they would die. She felt guilty about smoking crack, but the only time she felt she could face the world was when she was smoking. The problem, however, was the effect was so short, and the "down" that followed using was so low that she sometimes thought she would get the courage to kill herself when she was in one of the deep depressions that followed a cocaine run. In the 15 years, more or less, that Ms. D. had been using cocaine, she had had periods of abstinence, once up to a year, but went back to using again. Now, her pattern of using was two to three times per week.

The physical and psychiatric problems associated with cocaine use are numerous and potentially lethal. Ms. D.'s seriously pathologic pattern of use places her at high risk of both. It may be necessary for her to be removed from her environment to break the cycle of use she has established, as the lure to use will be so strong. A first question to ask is "do you go to it or does it come to you?" In other words, is the person who is supplying you with your drug bringing it to your home or do you have to go out to get it? If the former is the answer, the patient must go somewhere that the drug is not. Having to confront the drug being thrust into her face daily by someone insistent on selling it to her is going to make it extremely difficult for Ms. D. to stop using. This does not necessarily mean she must be in an institutional setting, although it may come to that. Being with friends or family who have no contact with the drug culture and can give her support for abstinence could be a first step.

Next, is the issue of whether to treat the depression. As discussed in the previous case, it is sometimes difficult to establish with certainty if depression is the result of the drug use or an independent entity. Many patients simply have no memory of a period of abstinence of sufficient length to know how they would feel without their chosen substance. In this case, however, the patient has had periods of clean time and still felt depressed. If no such clearcut history can be elicited, it is helpful for the clinician to know that the depression in the period after cocaine use typically resolves without treatment in 2 or 3 days. It must be stressed, however, that the depression during this period can be severe enough that hospitalization for safety may be necessary.

Once the decision is made to treat the depression, choosing the appropriate medication becomes something of a challenge. Concern has been raised that a combination of cocaine and TCA could increase the risk of seizures, although this concern appears to be more theoretic than real. Ciraulo et al. (28) do not report any cases of such. In fact, many clinicians in the early 1990s advocated the use of desipramine to counter cocaine craving. Although no good data support its usefulness in this regard, no untoward effects were reported (14–22). However, studies, not in humans, have shown that SSRI other than sertraline do increase the risk of seizure activity (23). Whether this occurs with humans is not known. Again, no reports of such are found.

As yet, no substantial information is found regarding the use of nefazodone or mirtazapine in this population, although some very preliminary but promising data are available on the use of venlafaxine. Thus, it appears that the safest method of treating Ms. D. at this time is with sertraline (Table 11-3).

CASE 11-4

Mary P. was proud of herself when, at 42 years of age, she recognized that she had developed a drinking problem, joined Alcoholics Anonymous, and successfully stopped using. Therefore, 20 years later, when she found she was unable to give up the hydrocodone she had been given after a hip replacement, it was all the more embarrassing and humbling for her to accept that once again she was powerless to control an addiction. The trouble was, although she accepted that she was dependent on the drug—she was taking three times as much as was prescribed— every time she tried to do something about it, she became depressed, cried constantly, could not concentrate, and thought about ending her life. She could not believe she loved the drug so much that just the idea of giving it up would make her want to end it all. Every attempt to walk away from it, however, seemed to make her feel that way. Besides, she was going to need help in overcoming her dependency on the drug. Mary had had one mild heart attack and her blood pressure, for which she took two types of medication, was somewhat erratic. She was afraid to try to stop without a doctor's help. She had already tried it twice and each time she did so, she experienced a gagging sensation in the back of her throat and a creepy feeling in her skin, accompanied by nausea and a deep aching in her back and joints. She really did not want to try stopping again without assistance.

Mary P. presents a particular challenge to the clinician. Her case involves issues regarding iatrogenic drug dependence, pain management, laws on the use of medications for detoxification from opiates, and the emergence of depressive symptoms with the removal of opiates. Each of these issues is discussed below.

First is the issue of iatrogenic substance dependence. Opiates are among the three most widely abused prescription drug categories in the country. Among individuals most likely to become addicted to such drugs are the elderly and women (24). In addition, some data suggest that a premorbid history of substance misuse also increases the risk that an individual will become iatrogenically addicted (25–27). Mary P. has all three risk factors.

The fact, however, is she legitimately had a need for analgesics and short-term administration of hydrocodone was reasonable just as would have been for any postoperative patient. The problem arose with the length of exposure and how the patient was able to escalate her dose without anyone noticing or questioning it. Clinicians increase the likelihood of iatrogenic drug misuse in the elderly by continuing to prescribe the drug beyond a typical length of time, not keeping an index of suspicious, and not questioning the need for continued use. Being an older woman, Mary was less likely to arouse the suspicion that she might be misusing her medications. Her excuse that she "lost" prescriptions or must have

Table 11-4. Cocaine use and depression (case 11-4)

Issue	Effects and How Addressed
Pain management	+/– of narcotics in nonterminal pain Improved analgesia with antidepressant Medication at lower doses of narcotics
Depression	Opioids known to act as antidepressant in some individuals Risk of interaction of selective serotonin reuptake inhibitors with tramadol
Detoxification	Referral to methadone clinic Hospitalization for inpatient detoxification Change to tramadol

misunderstood the instructions failed to arouse the suspicion that a young man saying the same thing might have. Physicians also promote substance misuse by writing for multiple refills or refilling prescriptions over the telephone without questioning whether such is really necessary. In addition, although we do not know if Mary was doing this, it is easy for older adults to "doctor shop." That is, they may see multiple doctors and obtain prescriptions for the same medication, thus making it possible to increase the amount of drug being taken.

Next is the issue of pain management. Does she still need something for analgesia? An in-depth discussion of the pros and cons of narcotic administration for nonterminal pain is beyond the scope of this book. Nevertheless, arguments occur on both sides of the debate. Regardless, if she does have ongoing pain, it is going to emerge strongly as her narcotics are reduced. She has also made it clear that when she reduces her medication, she becomes suicidally depressed. Observers have described this for many years, but it is not clear whether the individuals had a premorbid depression or not. Regardless, the depression emerges as the opiate is reduced or stopped.

The clinician might prepare the way for Mary to be detoxified by exploiting a property of TCA that would permit her to reduce her dose without experiencing withdrawal symptoms and at the same time experience relief of her depressive symptoms. Evidence suggests that the pain-relieving properties of morphine are enhanced by antidepressants including desipramine, amitriptyline, fluoxetine, and sertraline (28). It is also clear that some antidepressants (e.g., desipramine) can raise the levels of morphine and methadone by inhibiting their metabolism. Thus, a lower dose of the analgesic is needed to achieve the same level of pain relief. The clinician could begin to treat Mary's depression with one of these medications while decreasing the hydrocodone without her experiencing significant discomfort.

Now comes the more complex problem. As noted, opiate detoxification is a simple task. Simply placing an individual back on the dependent drug, spacing out the dosing and reducing the dose at each interval over time can accomplish the task nicely. For example, if Mary is taking 40 mg/day of hydrocodone, she could be placed on 10 mg every 6 hours, and the dose decreased by 2 mg at each dose to 8 mg every 6 hours. This could then be repeated every 5 to 7 days, first to 6 mg every 6 hours, then 4 mg every 6 hours, and so on and Mary would experience relatively little discomfort.

The problem is that this approach is illegal. The Federal Register clearly states that methadone is the only narcotic that can be used for the purpose of detoxification from or maintenance therapy of, opiate dependence. Further, this can take place only in the context of a federally, state, or locally licensed methadone program. Any licensed physician with a DEA number can prescribe opiates for pain relief, but not opiate maintenance or detoxification. Thus, the individual clinician who works outside of a methadone program and without a methadone license cannot use any scheduled drug for this purpose. A law has been passed that would provide for buprenorphine to be used for this purpose when and if it is permitted that a schedule III agent can be used for detoxification from opiates. As of this writing, however, this has not been done. Therefore, detoxification becomes more difficult in the face of medical problems and the patient's age.*

Given that Mary has labile hypertension, close monitoring of her blood pressure is indicated. The clonidine detoxification recipe given earlier could be risky because of the possibility of her blood pressure dropping precipitously, which increases the risk of an ischemic stroke or orthostatic hypertension with its attendant problem of falls or syncope. Inpatient detoxification would be the best choice, although few managed care companies would permit such in the absence of a clear and present significant health risk and no immediate problems exist.

One possible solution would be to refer Mary to a licensed methadone program for detoxification. Waiting lists for public programs tend to be fairly long in large cities, although private for-profit clinics typically work new patients in fairly quickly. Another problem arises in that not all towns or all states even have methadone programs available to them. Another possibility is to put Mary on tramadol, a mu agonist with reputedly low abuse potential (29). Although physiologic dependence can and does occur with tramadol use, especially among those, such as Mary, with a history of opiate dependence, it is not a scheduled drug and, therefore, can be used for detoxification (30). If the prescribing clinician keeps a close watch over the supply, just as with a benzodiazepine for alcohol withdrawal, this can be done safely and effectively.

If the tramadol approach is taken, much care must be exercised in the choice of antidepressant because toxic and lethal interactions have been reported between tramadol and SSRI (31–34). Once Mary is stable on her antidepressant, if an inpatient stay is not possible for detoxification, indications are to reduce the hydrocodone dose to the minimum necessary for pain relief, then a switch to tramadol. If this route is taken, the patient would need to be seen on a daily basis to have her vital signs taken, to be observed for signs of withdrawal, and to be evaluated regarding emergence or reemergence of depression.

Mary's situation is not a simple one. Hospitalization might eventually be required, even with very close monitoring, because of her age, medical conditions, and the possibility of medication interactions.

*Buprenorphine was approved for opiate dependence treatment in October of 2002.

REFERENCES

1. DiBari M, Silvestrini G, Chiarlone M, et al. Features of excessive alcohol drinking in older adults distinctively captured by behavioral and biological screening instruments: an epidemiological study. *J Clin Epidemiol* 2002;55(1):41–47.
2. Clay SW. Comparison of AUDIT and CAGE questionnaire in screening for alcohol use disorders in elderly primary care outpatients. *J Am Osteopath Assoc* 1997;97(10):588–592.
3. Affairs AMCoS. Alcoholism in the elderly: Council report. *JAMA* 1996;275(10):797–801.
4. Oslin DW, Katz IR, Edell WS, et al. Effects of alcohol consumption on the treatment of depression among elderly patients. *Am J Geriatr Psychiatry* 2000;8(3):215–220.

5. McGrath PJ, Nunes EV, Stewart JW, et al. Imipramine treatment of alcoholics with primary depression: a placebo controlled clinical trial. *Arch Gen Psychiatry* 1996;535(3):232–240.

6. Hyatt MC, Bird MA. Amitriptyline augments and prolongs ethanol induced euphoria. *J Clin Psychopharmacol* 1987;7:277–278.

7. Ciraulo DA. Clinical pharmacokinetics of imipramine and desipramine in alcoholics and normal volunteers. *Clin Pharmacol Ther* 1988;43:509.

8. Cornelius JR, Sallou IM, Ehler JG, et al. Fluoxetine in depressed alcoholics: a double blind, placebo controlled trial. *Arch Gen Psychiatry* 1997;54(8):700–705.

9. Neylan TC, Reynolds III CF, Kupfer DJ. Neuropsychiatric aspects of sleep and sleep disorders. In: Yudovsky SC, Hales RE, eds. *The American Psychiatric Press textbook of neuropsychiatry.* Washington, DC: American Psychiatric Press, 1997.

10. Haney M, Ward AS, Comer SD, et al. Bupropion SR worsens mood during marijuana withdrawal in humans. *Psychopharmacology* 2001;155(2):171–179.

11. Lee EW, D'Alonzo GE. Cigarette smoking, nicotine addiction, and its pharmacologic treatment. *Arch Intern Med* 1993;153(1):34–48.

12. Prochazka AV, Petty TL, Nett L, et al. Transdermal clonidine reduced some withdrawal symptoms but did not increase smoking cessation. *Arch Intern Med* 1992;152(10):2065–2069.

13. Sees KL, Stalcup SA. Combining clonidine and nicotine replacement for treatment of nicotine withdrawal. *J Psychoactive Drugs* 1989;21(3):355–359.

14. Campbell JL, Thomas HM, Gabrielli W, et al. Impact of desipramine or carbamazepine on patient retention in outpatient cocaine treatment: preliminary findings. *J Addict Dis* 1994;13(4):191–199.

15. Hall SM, Tunis S, Triffleman E, et al. Continuity of care and desipramine in primary cocaine abusers. *J Nerv Ment Dis* 1994;182(10):570–575.

16. Kaminer Y. Desipramine facilitation of cocaine abstinence in an adolescent. *J Am Acad Child Adolesc Psychiatry* 1992;31(2):312–317.

17. Kolar AF, Brown BS, Weddington WW, et al. Treatment of cocaine dependence in methadone maintenance clients: a pilot study comparing the efficacy of desipramine and amantadine. *International Journal of the Addictions* 1992;27(7):849–868.

18. Kosten TR, Morgan CM, Flacione J, et al. Pharmacotherapy for cocaine abusing methadone maintained patients using amantadine or desipramine. *Arch Gen Psychiatry* 1992;49(11):894–898.

19. Tennant FS, Rawson RA. Cocaine and amphetamine dependence treated with desipramine. *NIDA Res Monogr* 1983;43:351–355.

20. Weddington WW Jr., Brown BS, Haertzen CA, et al. Comparison of amantadine and desipramine combined with psychotherapy for treatment of cocaine dependence. *Am J Drug Alcohol Abuse* 1991;17(2):137–152.

21. Covi L, Montory ID, Hess J, et al. Double blind comparison of desipramine and placebo for treatment of cocaine dependence. *Clin Pharmacol Ther* 1994;55:132.

22. Nelson RA, Gorelick DA, Keenan RM, et al. Cardiovascular interactions of desipramine, fluoxetine, and cocaine in cocaine dependent outpatients. *Am J Addict* 1996;5(4):321–326.

23. O'Dell LE, George FR, Ritz MC. Antidepressant drugs appear to enhance cocaine induced toxicity. *Exp Clin Psychopharmacol* 2000;8(1):133–141.

24. Abuse NIoD. *Prescription drugs: abuse and addiction*. Bethesda, MD: National Institutes of Health, 2002.

25. Oswald LM, Roache JD, Rhoades HM. Predictors of individual differences in alprazolam self-medication. *Exp Clin Psychopharmacol* 1999;74:379–390.

26. Sproule BA, Bsto UE, Somer G, et al. Characteristics of dependent and non-dependent regular users of codeine. *J Clin Psychopharmacol* 1999;19(4):367–372.

27. Chabal C, Erjavec MK, Jacobson L, et al. Prescription opiate abuse in chronic pain patients: clinical criteria, incidence and predictors. *Clin J Pain* 1997;13(2):150–155.

28. Ciraulo DA, Creelman WL, Shader RI, et al. Cyclic antidepressants. In: Ciraulo DA, Shader RI, Greenblatt DJ, et al., eds. *Drug interactions in psychiatry,* 2nd ed. Baltimore: Williams & Wilkins, 1995:430.

29. Desmeules JA. The tramadol option. *Eur J Pain* 2000;4(Suppl A): 15–21.

30. Liu Z, Zhou WH, Lian Z, et al. Drug dependence and abuse potential of tramadol. *Acta Pharmacol Sin* 1999;20(1):52–54.

31. Gonzalez-Pinto A, Imaz H, De Heredia JL, et al. Mania and tramadol-fluoxetine combination. *Am J Psychiatry* 2001;158(6): 964–965.

32. Ripple MG, Pestaner JP, Levine BS, et al. Lethal combination of tramadol and multiple drugs affecting serotonin. *Am J Forensic Med Pathol* 2000;21(4):370–374.

33. Lantz MS, Buchalter EN, Giambanco V. Serotonin syndrome following the administration of tramadol with paroxetine. *Int J Geriatr Psychiatry* 1998;13(5):343–353.

34. Mason BJ, Blackburn KH. Possible serotonin syndrome associated with tramadol and sertraline coadministration. *Ann Pharmacother* 1997;31(2):175–177.

Anxiety Disorders

1. The anxiety disorders are presented
   a. Social anxiety disorder: more common in women, onset in teens
   b. Simple phobia: also more common in women, onset in teens
   c. Obsessive compulsive disorder: slight female preponderance
   d. Posttraumatic stress disorder: slight female preponderance
   e. Generalized anxiety disorder: has been a controversial diagnosis
   f. Panic disorder: can be associated with agoraphobia
   g. Anxiety caused by a general medical condition, acute stress disorder, and substance-induced anxiety disorder: relatively new diagnoses to the *Diagnostic and Statistical Manual of Mental Disorders,* data just accumulating
2. Comorbidity is high and differs by specific diagnosis
   a. Nicotine: can have a paradoxical calming effect when individual is anxious
   b. Alcohol: decreases severity of panic in panic disorder; not necessarily helps social phobia
   c. Cocaine: use widespread among those with posttraumatic stress disorder as it is among others
   d. Opiates: incidence of panic disorder increasing among methadone maintenance patients
3. Medication issues
   a. Benzodiazepines widely used: relatively contraindicated in addicted population
   b. Interaction of various drugs and medications

BACKGROUND

The anxiety disorders, a group of nine psychiatric conditions, together are more common than the other psychiatric disorders, surpassing even affective disorders in frequency of occurrence. Together, anxiety disorders afflict more than 25% of the population at some time in their lives (1,2). Although each is a distinct entity, the anxiety disorders frequently co-occur with each other and with both mood disorders and substance use disorders. The anxiety disorders are panic disorder with or without agoraphobia, specific phobia, social anxiety, obsessive compulsive disorder (OCD), posttraumatic stress disorder (PTSD), generalized anxiety disorder (GAD), anxiety caused by a general medical condition, acute stress disorder, and substance-induced anxiety disorder. The latter three conditions are relative newcomers to the *Diagnostic and Statistical Manual of Mental Disorders* (DSM) and fewer data are available about them, medication responses to them, and comorbidity. Therefore, discussion in this and the next chapter focuses on the first six conditions, about which more is known. Both psychiatric and physiologic responses, notably hyperactivity of the sympathetic nervous system, are prominent features of the anxiety disorders. The cause of such symptoms varies, depending on the exact disorder.

Although placed together categorically, the cause of the anxiety disorders and their prognoses vary widely.

DISORDERS

Social anxiety disorder is the most common of the disorders, with a lifetime prevalence rate variably estimated at 3% to 13%. It involves the onset of feelings of anxiety about meeting new people, public speaking, and other similar social events. The disorder occurs slightly more often among women than men (1.4:1), with the median age of onset being 16 years. Factors predicting the occurrence of social phobia include lower education, lower income, and never having been married (3–6).

Specific or simple phobia is a fear or anxiety reaction caused by the presence of a feared subject. Examples include a fear of spiders, of high places, and of being in confined spaces. Lifetime prevalence is variably given as being from 6.5% to 20% and, as with social phobia, is more common among women than men (3.8:1), with onset at about age 15 years (4).

Obsessive–Compulsive Disorder

Obsessive–compulsive disorder (OCD) is a condition in which obsessive thoughts about situations, subjects, or persons predominate. Those with OCD often engage in compulsive behaviors whose purpose is to "undo" or compensate for the obsessions. Lifetime prevalence, according to studies here and elsewhere, is about 2.5%. In adult onset, most studies show a slight female preponderance (~55% female), but a male preponderance in child and adolescent onset populations (65%). Most cases begin in the late teens and twenties, whereas onset after 50 years of age is uncommon (7).

Posttraumatic Stress Disorder

Posttraumatic stress disorder (PTSD) is an anxiety disorder that occurs in response to overwhelming trauma outside of the realm of normal human experience. Such can occur in the context of rape, witnessing a murder, or of being exposed to war and other violence. Lifetime prevalence of PTSD ranges from 1% to 15% and occurs slightly more often among women than men (8,9).

Generalized Anxiety Disorder

A diagnosis of generalized anxiety disorder (GAD) has generated controversy among researchers; some describe it as a component of other anxiety disorders, rather than being a diagnosis in and of itself. It is characterized by excessive worry of a chronic nature in conjunction with somatic complaints. Lifetime prevalence of this disorder is 5% and is over represented among women by approximately 2:1. Unemployment and being separated, widowed, or divorced are all risk factors for developing GAD (10–12).

Panic Disorder

Panic disorder, with or without agoraphobia, is a condition characterized by the occurrence of panic attacks. These are discrete episodes during which feelings of fear or general discomfort and negative anticipation predominate. Each is associated with a number of physiologic symptoms including, but not limited to, cardiac palpitations, shortness of breath, numbness or tingling sensations, and fear of "going crazy" or of being "out of control." Such episodes are time-limited and can occur at seemingly random intervals, or when exposed to or in anticipation of specific events or experiences. Individuals with panic disorder may become increasingly restricted in their activities, becoming anxious at the risk of having panic attacks (anticipatory anxiety). With onset typically in young adulthood, panic disorder starts later than others of the anxiety disorders. However, as with other anxiety disorders, panic disorder tends to be diagnosed more often among women and lifetime prevalence is about 1.5% to 3% (13).

Agoraphobia

Agoraphobia, a fear of open places, takes its name from the Greek "agora," meaning market. Lifetime prevalence of the disorder is 3% to 6.7%, with occurrence in women more than twice that of men (2.2:1). Unlike social and simple phobias, median age of onset of agoraphobia is in the late twenties. The National Comorbidity Study shows the disorder to be disproportionately higher among blacks and among individuals with little education and lower income (4). Individuals with agoraphobia become increasingly restricted in the area in which they are comfortable. They may not be able to leave their neighborhood, block, yard, or house without suffering a panic attack, depending on their particular zone of comfort (Table 12-1).

Comorbidity

Anxiety is greater among persons who misuse substances than among the general population, regardless of the drug of choice. In one study, for example, 26% of all substance-dependent individuals surveyed met criteria for PTSD (14). More than 14% of individuals with OCD have comorbid substance dependence (15). As is often the case with psychiatric conditions and substance misuse, however, it is often difficult to discern which is primary and which secondary. Some substances of abuse or their withdrawal can cause anxiety reactions, whereas some individuals suffering from anxiety will find temporary relief of their symptoms by using the various substances (16). Individuals suffering from most primary anxiety disorders are at an increased risk of developing additional anxiety disorders, mood disorders, and substance use disorders. Some debate whether individuals with social phobia are more susceptible to abusive use of alcohol (17–19). It is important to note that, whereas the anxiety disorders by themselves may not increase the risk of suicide, when combined with substance misuse, suicide can be a significant danger (20).

Nicotine

As is the case with depression, anxiety disorders are prevalent among individuals with nicotine dependence (21,22). Estimates are that 10% to 15% of this population has some anxiety disorder at any given time (23). Further, in nicotine-dependent persons, nicotine has a seemingly paradoxic effect of producing a calming effect when the individual is anxious (24,25).

Alcohol

Alcohol use is widespread, and higher among those with anxiety disorders than among the general population. It is so common, in fact, that one researcher commented ". . . . the presence of an anxiety disorder predicts the presence of alcohol dependence and vice versa . . ." (23,26). Although anxiety symptoms may decrease with

Table 12-1. Anxiety disorders

Disorder	Percent Population (Lifetime)	Male:Female	Onset	Predictors
Panic disorder with or without agoraphobia	1.5–3	M < F	Onset in young adulthood	
Specific phobia	6.5–20	1:3.8	15 years of age	Lower social and economic status, lower income
Social phobia	3–13	1:1.4	16 years of age	Higher in female and in previously married
Obsessive compulsive disorder	1.9–2.5	Slight female preponderance with adult onset	Late teens, early twenties	
Posttraumatic stress disorder	1.5–15	5% to 10.4%		Male: combat exposure and witness Female: rape and sexual molestation
Generalized anxiety disorder	5.7	1:2	Onset in childhood or adolescence rare	>24 years of age, separated, widowed, divorced, unemployed, a homemaker

detoxification, they do not disappear, a fact that has some prognostic significance. Individuals who continue to experience significant anxiety are at risk of early relapse to drinking, making it important for the treating clinician to continue to monitor these symptoms and treat such if they persist (27). Panic disorder, in particular, appears frequently among those with alcoholism. It is possible, but not definite, that alcohol may decrease the frequency and severity of panic symptoms (28–30).

Where social phobia and alcohol occur concomitantly, research suggests the anxiety is more likely to have preceded the drinking, suggesting self-medication (31). One group looked at what social phobics who drank alcohol might be hoping to gain from alcohol use. They found that alcohol did not decrease physiologic symptoms of anxiety. However, when subjects thought they were drinking alcohol and believed it would relieve their anxiety, they did, in fact, show improvement in their anxiety symptoms (32).

Posttraumatic stress disorder is also highly associated with alcohol use disorders, especially in women, who show a threefold increase in such (8,33). Likewise, panic disorder, OCD, and GAD are all highly associated with alcohol misuse. The relationship with social phobia, however, is not as clearly defined (4,34–37).

Cannabis

The literature has many reports of the onset of panic attacks with and without agoraphobia occurring in the context of cannabis use. In some cases, the anxiety disorder continued even after cessation of cannabis use (38–41). Although experimentation with marijuana can be as common among patients with anxiety disorder as among the general population, some suggest that continued use, at least among those with panic disorder, may be the exception rather than the rule. Cannabis appears to induce anxiety reactions in this population and individuals for whom this happens tend to stop using because of the discomfort it causes (42).

Cocaine

It is not uncommon for anxiety symptoms to occur as a result of cocaine use. Panic disorder, in particular, has been reported among cocaine users (43–45). An increased incidence of PTSD is found among cocaine users as well. One study of individuals seeking treatment for their addiction found that as many as 20% of cocaine addicts met criteria for PTSD, with the PTSD predating the substance use (46,47). The presence of the anxiety disorder, however, does not appear to predict ongoing use (48). Abstinence from cocaine helps to decrease some of the PTSD symptoms, although many patients continue to have intrusive thoughts (49). Further, memories of traumatic events tend to increase craving for cocaine and appear to be strong cues for relapse to cocaine use (50).

Opioids

Estimates are that more than 50% of patients on methadone maintenance have at least one anxiety disorder (51). PTSD, for example, is prevalent. As many as 20% of women and 11% of men may meet the diagnostic criteria for this disorder (47,52). It also appears that panic attacks among patients in methadone maintenance clinics are common and increasing in frequency. In the early 1980s, panic attacks were found to occur in 1% of the population. By the early 1990s, the percentage rose to 13%, likely as a direct result of cocaine use (53). In addition, many observers have pointed out the obsessive quality of heroin use. Estimate is that, among such users, the full diagnosis of OCD is present in approximately 11% of cases—more than four times that of the general population (20).

Effects on Medications

Benzodiazepines, a popular class of drugs, have been a mainstay of treatment for anxiety disorders. They are also among the most abused of all prescription drugs in the United States (54). Further, this class of drugs may be abused by as many as 40% of substance abusers seeking treatment (55). Because of their popularity among individuals who abuse a variety of drugs, how best to treat individuals with comorbid substance and anxiety disorders poses a particular problem for the treatment provider.

Considerable concern exists that individuals with substance use disorders and anxiety should not be treated with benzodiazepines because of the belief that (a) these drugs would act as a trigger for resumption of use and (b) substance abusers are at a high risk of benzodiazepine abuse. In addition, especially among veterans with PTSD, there is particular concern regarding the possible emergence of violent dyscontrol problems if this population were exposed to this class of drugs. Although the evidence has not consistently supported an absolute prohibition against treating persons who misuse substances with benzodiazepines, the prevailing wisdom is to do so only with great caution and as briefly as possible (56–60).

Nicotine can increase clearance of benzodiazepines and of imipramine so that more of these medications will be needed to adequately treat smokers for their anxiety (61). Individuals with alcohol problems preferentially gravitate toward benzodiazepines, if given access to such (62). Alcohol in combination with benzodiazepines results in an additive decrease in performance on cognitive and skills testing (63,64). Further, alcohol in combination with alprazolam, possibly as a result of disinhibition, has been found to be associated with an increase in aggression (65). Buspirone in combination with alcohol has an additive sedative effect but does not affect performance or increase aggression as does alprazolam (63).

Clomipramine, commonly prescribed for OCD, when combined with alcohol has more than an additive effect on performance of motor skills and cognitive functioning (66).

Benzodiazepine abuse is common among opiate-dependent individuals in methadone maintenance programs (67). This class of drugs has been used for a number of years to augment narcotics for medical management of pain, but in controlled environments. The potential for respiratory suppression and death with this combination is a concern in the nonhospitalized patient. Reports are found in the literature of deaths from opiate—benzodiazepine combinations (68,69).

Much evidence shows that social phobia, OCD, GAD, and panic disorder are well treated and possibly best treated over the long term with antidepressants, including the serotonin reuptake inhibitors, tricyclics, and venlafaxine, which may speak to the lack of necessity of treating these conditions with potentially addictive drugs (70,71). However, the caveats noted for each of these medications in conjunction with substances of abuse then become applicable in these cases (Table 12-2).

Table 12-2. Anxiety disorder and comorbidity

	Incidence and Effect with Anxiety Disorder	Medication Effects
Nicotine	Much increased: generally has a calming effect in nicotine-dependent individuals	Can reduce concentrations of imipramine and benzodiazepines so that more will be necessary to be effective
Alcohol	Increased with most; question with social phobia; much increased with females with PTSD Continued anxiety after detox Often a relapse cue ↑ With PD Alcohol → ↓ frequency and severity of attacks	Can prolong effects of some benzodiazepines; with high dose of benzodiazepines in combination can be fatal
Marijuana	May precipitate anxiety: if does, use is self-limited	
Cocaine	Increased anxiety among cocaine users, high incidence of PTSD among cocaine users Abstinence→↓some PTSD symptoms but memories of trauma ↑↑↑ craving	Tricyclic: cocaine interaction → additive cardiotoxicity and ↑ risk of seizure activity
Heroin/opioids	Higher incidence of anxiety symptoms among heroin users; increasing because of cocaine Increased incidence of PTSD Increased incidence of OCD	Combination of some benzodiazepines and opiates can be fatal

OCD, obsessive-compulsive disorder; PD, panic disorder; PTSD, posttraumatic stress disorder.

REFERENCES

1. Brawman-Mintzer O, ed. *Generalized anxiety disorder.* Philadelphia: WB Saunders, 2001.
2. Ninan PT. Recent perspectives on the diagnosis and treatment of generalized anxiety disorder. *American Journal of Managed Care* 2001;7(Suppl 11):S367–S376.
3. Pollack MH. Comorbidity, neurobiology, and pharmacotherapy of social anxiety disorder. *J Clin Psychiatry* 2001;62(Suppl 12):24–29.
4. Magee W, Eaton J, William W, et al. Agoraphobia, simple phobia, and social phobia in the National Comorbidity Survey. *Arch Gen Psychiatry* 1996;53(2):159–168.
5. den Boer JA. Social anxiety disorder/social phobia: epidemiology, diagnosis, neurobiology, and treatment. *Compr Psychiatry* 2000; 41(6):405–415.
6. Juster HR, Heimberg RG. Social phobia: longitudinal course and long-term outcome of cognitive-behavioral treatment. *Psychiatr Clin North Am* 1995;18:821–842.
7. Antony MM, Downie F, Swinson RP. Diagnostic issues and epidemiology in obsessive–compulsive disorder. In: Swinson RP, Antony MM, Rachman S, eds. *Obsessive–compulsive disorder: theory, research, and treatment.* New York: Guilford Press, 1998.
8. Kessler RC, Sonnega A, Bromet E, et al. Posttraumatic stress disorder in the National Comorbidity Survey. *Arch Gen Psychiatry* 1995;52(12):1048–1060.
9. Helzer JE, Robins LN, McEvoy L. Posttraumatic stress disorder in the general population. *N Engl J Med* 1987;317:1630–1634.
10. Schweizer E. Generalized anxiety disorder: longitudinal course and pharmacologic treatment. *Psychiatr Clin North Am* 1995;18: 843–857.
11. Wittchen HU, Zhao S, Kessler RC, et al. DSM-III-R generalized anxiety disorder in the National Comorbidity Survey. *Arch Gen Psychiatry* 1994;51(5):355–364.
12. Woodman CL, Noyes RJ, Black DW, et al. A five-year follow-up study of generalized anxiety disorder and panic disorder. *J Nerv Ment Dis* 1999;187(1):3–9.
13. Weissman MM, Bland RC, Canino GJ, et al. The cross national epidemiology of panic disorder. *Arch Gen Psychiatry* 1997;54(4): 305–309.
14. Teegen F, Zumbeck S. Prevalence of traumatic experiences and posttraumatic stress disorder in substance dependent persons: an explorative study. *Psychotherapeutisch* 2000;45(1):44–49.
15. Antony MM, Downie F, Swinson RP. Diagnostic issues and epidemiology in obsessive compulsive disorder. In: Swinson RP, Antony MM, Rachman S, et al. *Obsessive compulsive disorder: theory, research and treatment.* New York: Guilford Press, 1998: 3–32.
16. Walfish S, Massey R, Krone A. Anxiety and anger among abusers of different substances. *Drug Alcohol Depend* 1990;25(3):253–256.
17. Merikangas KR, Whitaker A, Angst J, et al. Comorbidity and boundaries of affective disorders with anxiety disorders and substance misuse: results of an international task force. *Br J Psychiatry* 1996;168(Suppl 30):58–67.
18. Crum RM, Pratt LA. Risk of heavy drinking and alcohol use disorders in social phobia: a prospective analysis. *Am J Psychiatry* 2001;158(10):1693–1700.

19. Merikangas KR, Angst J. Comorbidity and social phobia: evidence from clinical, epidemiologic, and genetic studies. *Eur Arch Psychiatry Clin Neurosci* 1995;244(6):297–303.

20. Friedman S, Smith L, Fogel A. Suicidality in panic disorder: a comparison with schizophrenic, depressed, and other anxiety disorder outpatients. *J Anxiety Disord* 1999;13(5):447–461.

21. Breslau N, Kilbey MM, Andreski P. Nicotine dependence, major depression, and anxiety in young adults. *Arch Gen Psychiatry* 1991;48(12):1069–1074.

22. Kirch DG. Nicotine and major mental disorders. In: Piasecki M, Newhouse PA, eds. *Nicotine in psychiatry: psychopathology and emerging therapeutics.* Washington, DC: American Psychiatric Press, 2000:111–130.

23. Farrell M, Howes S, Bebbington P, et al. Nicotine, alcohol and drug dependence and psychiatric comorbidity: results of a national household survey. *Br J Psychiatry* 2001;179:432–437.

24. Grobe JE, Perkins KA. Behavioral factors influencing the effects of nicotine. In: Piasecki M, Newhouse PA, eds. *Nicotine in psychiatry: psychopathology and emerging therapeutics.* Washington, DC: American Psychiatry Press, 2000:59–82.

25. Juliano LM, Brandon TH. Effects of nicotine dose, instructional set, and outcome expectancies on the subjective effects of smoking in the presence of a stressor. *J Abnorm Psychol* 2002;111(1):89–97.

26. Kushner MG, Sher KJ, Erickson DJ. Prospective analysis of the relation between DSM-III anxiety disorders and alcohol use disorders. *Am J Psychiatry* 1999;156(5):723–732.

27. Driessen M, Meier S, Hill A, et al. The course of anxiety, depression and drinking behaviors after completed detoxification in alcoholics with and without comorbid anxiety and depressive disorders. *Alcohol Alcohol* 2001;36(3):249–255.

28. Kushner MG, Mackenzie TB, Fiszdon J, et al. The effects of alcohol consumption on laboratory induced panic and state anxiety. *Arch Gen Psychiatry* 1996;53(3):264–270.

29. Lepola U. Alcohol and depression in panic disorder. *Acta Psychiatr Scand Suppl* 1994;377:33–35.

30. George DT, Lindquist T, Ragan PW, et al. Effect of alcoholism on the incidence of lactate induced panic attacks. *Biol Psychiatry* 1997;42(11):992–999.

31. Merikangas KR, Stevens DE, Fenton B, et al. Co-morbidity and familial aggregation of alcoholism and anxiety disorders. *Psychol Med* 1998;28(4):773–788.

32. Himle JA, Abelson JL, Haghightgou H, et al. Effect of alcohol on social phobic anxiety. *Am J Psychiatry.* 1999;156(8):1237–1243.

33. Breslau N, Davis GC, Peterson EL, Schultz L. Psychiatric sequelae of posttraumatic stress disorder in women. *Arch Gen Psychiatry* 1997;54:81–87.

34. Rodgers B, Korten AE, Jorm AF, et al. Non linear relationships in associations of depression and anxiety with alcohol use. *Psychol Med* 2000;30(2):421–423.

35. Regier DA, Farmer ME, Rae DS, et al. Comorbidity of mental disorders with alcohol and other drug abuse: results from the Epidemiological Catchment Area study. *JAMA* 1990;264(19):2511–2518.

36. Helzer J, Pryzbeck T. The co-occurrence of alcoholism with other psychiatric disorders in the general population and its impact on treatment. *J Stud Alcohol* 1988;49:219–224.

37. Grant BF, Harford TC, Dawson DA. Prevalence of DSM-IV alcohol abuse and dependence: United States, 1992. *Alcohol Health and Research World* 1994;18(3):243–248.
38. Langs G, Fabisch H, Fabisch K, et al. Can cannabis trigger recurrent panic attacks in susceptible patients? *Eur Psychiatry* 1997;12(8):415–419.
39. Deas D, Gerding L, Hazy J. Marijuana and panic disorder. *J Am Acad Child Adolesc Psychiatry* 2000;39(12):1467.
40. Moran C. Depersonalization and agoraphobia associated with marijuana use. *Br J Med Psychol* 1986;59(Part 2):187–196.
41. Strohle A, Muller M, Rupprecht R. Marijuana precipitation of panic disorder with agoraphobia. *Acta Psychiatr Scand* 1998;98(3):254–255.
42. Szuster RR, Pontius EB, Campos PE. Marijuana sensitivity and panic anxiety. *J Clin Psychiatry* 1988;49(11):427–429.
43. Geracioti TD, Post RM. Onset of panic disorder associated with rare use of cocaine. *Biol Psychiatry* 1991;29(4):403–406.
44. Louie AK, Lannon RA, Ketter TA. Treatment of cocaine induced panic disorder. *Am J Psychiatry* 1989;146(1):40–44.
45. Price WA, Giannini AJ. Phencyclidine and "crack" precipitated panic disorder. *Am J Psychiatry* 1987;144(5):686–687.
46. Najavits LM, Gastfirend DR, Barber JP, et al. Cocaine dependence with and without PTSD among subjects in the National Institute on Drug Abuse Collaborative Cocaine Treatment study. *Am J Psychiatry* 1998;155(2):214–219.
47. Cottler LB, Compton WM, Mager D, et al. Posttraumatic stress disorder among substance users from the general population. *Am J Psychiatry* 1993;149(5):664–670.
48. Wasserman DA, Havassy BE, Boles SM. Traumatic events and posttraumatic stress disorder in cocaine users entering private treatment. *Drug Alcohol Depend* 1997;46:1–8.
49. Dansky BS, Brady KT, Saladin ME. Untreated symptoms of PTSD among cocaine-dependent individuals: changes over time. *J Subst Abuse Treat* 1998;15(6):499–504.
50. Coffey SF, Saladin M, Drobes DJ, et al. Trauma and substance cue reactivity in individuals with comorbid posttraumatic stress disorder and cocaine or alcohol dependence. *Drug Alcohol Depend* 2002;65(2):115–127.
51. Milby JB, Sims MK, Khuder SS, et al. Psychiatric comorbidity: prevalence in methadone maintenance treatment. *Am J Drug Alcohol Abuse* 1996;22(1):95–107.
52. Villagomez RE, Meyer TJ, Lin MM, et al. Posttraumatic stress disorder among inner city methadone maintenance patients. *J Subst Abuse Treat* 1995;12(4):253–257.
53. Rosen MI, Kosten TR. Cocaine associated panic attacks in methadone maintained patients. *Am J Drug Alcohol Abuse* 1992;18(1):57–62.
54. Abuse NIoD. *Prescription drugs: abuse and addiction.* Bethesda, MD: National Institutes of Health, 2002.
55. Malcolm R, Brady KT, Johnston AL, et al. Types of benzodiazepines abused by chemically dependent inpatients. *J Psychoactive Drugs* 1993;25(4):314–319.
56. Nunes EV, McGrath PJ, Quitkin FM. Treating anxiety in patients with alcoholism. *J Clin Psychiatry* 1995;56(Suppl 2):3–9.

57. Ross J, Darke S. The nature of benzodiazepine dependence among heroin users in Sydney, Australia. *Addiction* 2000;95(12): 1785–1793.

58. Kosten TR, Fontana A, Sernyak MJ, et al. Benzodiazepine use in posttraumatic stress disorder among veterans with substance abuse. *J Nerv Ment Dis* 2000;188(7):454–459.

59. Chilcoat HD, Breslau N. Posttraumatic stress disorder and drug disorders: testing causal pathways. *Arch Gen Psychiatry* 1998; 55(10):913–917.

60. Ciraulo DA, Nace EP. Benzodiazepine treatment of anxiety or insomnia in substance abuse patients. *Am J Addict* 2000;9(4): 276–284.

61. Ciraulo DA, Shader RI, Greenblatt DJ, et al., eds. *Drug interactions in psychiatry.* Baltimore, MD: Williams & Wilkins, 1995.

62. de Wit H, Doty P. Preference for ethanol and diazepam in light and moderate social drinkers: a within subjects study. *Psychopharmacology* 1994;115(4):529–538.

63. Rush CR, Griffitchs RR. Acute participant-rated and behavioral effects of alprazolam and buspirone, alone and in combination with ethanol, in normal volunteers. *Exp Clin Psychopharmacol* 1997;5(1):28–36.

64. Nichols JM, Martin F, Kirkby KC. A comparison of the effect of lorazepam on memory in heavy and low social drinkers. *Psychopharmacology* 1993;112(4):475–482.

65. Bond AJ, Silveira JC. The combination of alprazolam and alcohol on behavioral aggression. *J Stud Alcohol* 1993;(Suppl):30–39.

66. Berlin I, Cournot A, Zimmer R, et al. Evaluation and comparison of the interaction between alcohol and moclobemide or clomipramine in healthy subjects. *Psychopharmacology* 1990;100(1):40–45.

67. DuPont RL, Saylor KE. Marijuana and benzodiazepines in patients receiving methadone treatment. *JAMA* 1989;261(16):3409.

68. Gilliland HE, Prasad BK, Mirakhur RK, et al. An investigation of the potential morphine sparing effect of midazolam. *Anaesthesia* 1997;51(9):808–811.

69. Patterson DR, Ptacek JT, Carrougher GJ, et al. Lorazepam as an adjunct to opioid analgesics in the treatment of burn pain. *Pain* 1997;72(3):367–374.

70. Keller MB. The long-term clinical course of generalized anxiety disorder. *J Clin Psychiatry* 2002;63(Suppl 8):11–16.

71. Gorman JM. Treatment of generalized anxiety disorder. *J Clin Psychiatry* 2002;63(Suppl 8):17–23.

Treatment of Anxiety Disorders and Substance Misuse

1. Social anxiety disorder and alcohol
   a. Social anxiety not really improved with alcohol, although high incidence of comorbidity
   b. Risk factors for later alcohol problems are reviewed: early onset of drinking, male gender, relative nonresponse to effects of alcohol
   c. Medication choices reviewed
      i. Buspirone not effective against this disorder
      ii. Benzodiazepines offer some short-term benefit but very temporary; debatable whether this can legitimately be offered to someone with a substance use disorder
      iii. Serotonin reuptake inhibitors are considered first-line therapy
      iv. Disulfiram and naltrexone can help to deter individual from drinking
      v. Patients need to change their milieu in order to decrease likelihood of relapse
2. Posttraumatic stress disorder and cocaine
   a. Comorbidity between the two commonly occurs
   b. Increase in symptoms of posttraumatic stress disorder common in early abstinence period
   c. Flashbacks: common relapse cue
   d. Therapist and patient must balance dealing with issues and learning relapse prevention skills before delving too deeply into issues with individual with comorbid posttraumatic stress disorder and substance misuse
   e. Medication alternatives
      i. Sertraline likely best choice
      ii. No indication for antipsychotics in such cases
      iii. Benzodiazepines, at most, temporarily
3. Panic disorder, marijuana, and alcohol
   a. Cannabis can precipitate onset of panic attacks
      i. Panic sufferers typically stop using marijuana spontaneously
      ii. Panic attacks may not stop with ceasing cannabis use
   b. Alcohol relieves symptoms of panic
      i. Fact of rapid relief makes intervention difficult
      ii. Patient must learn relaxation techniques while trying to achieve abstinence, relapse rate high
   c. Medication alternatives; serotonin reuptake inhibitors preferred

CASE 13-1

Tom, now 43, started drinking in high school. It was the only way he could get up the courage to talk to people. Dating was a terrifying prospect. If it hadn't been for friends setting him up, he probably would never have gone out with the girl he ended up marrying. When he was getting his business degree, it didn't occur to him that he was going to have to entertain company clients, or worse, that he would have to get up in front of groups and make presentations. Fortunately, it was always acceptable to have a beer or two or a glass of wine at business gatherings, and that helped a lot toward calming his nerves. Besides, he could handle it—he was never really drunk. The problem was, however, over time, his "nerves" seemed to be bothering him more and more. He really needed a drink at noon just to keep down his anxiety, which seemed to be worsening as the years went by. When he woke up one morning with his heart racing and reached for a beer instead of a cup of coffee, he knew he was in trouble.

Tom's case illustrates more than one aspect of anxiety and alcohol use. As noted in Chapter 12, Tom is not unique among individuals with social phobia in that his belief that alcohol will improve his ability to perform, to get up in a crowd and speak, did, in fact, make it happen. In addition, he follows a predictable pattern for the individual expected to develop significant drinking problems: male, early onset of use, little response to heavy drinking compared with others, progressing to day time use. He gravitated to an environment in which his use would be overlooked because he could blend into the crowd as well. Drinkers tend to find the company of drinkers, and this is exactly what Tom has done.

Before anything else can be done, this patient has to be detoxified from alcohol. Any patient who needs an "eye-opener" (a drink first thing in the morning to counter the effects of withdrawal) also needs help with withdrawal and medical monitoring. The decision hints in Chapter 5 should be applied in this case to determine the environment in which detoxification should take place.

As discussed, it is anticipated that withdrawal will take 5 to 7 days, with the peak of symptoms occurring about 48 to 72 hours after he stops or seriously curtails his alcohol use. Tremulousness, anxiety, and discomfort during this period should not be interpreted as anything other than withdrawal (i.e., should not be construed as anxiety).

Once the patient has been safely detoxified, stable, and back into his typical environment, his issues of social phobia can be addressed. Much more needs to be known about Tom and what is required of him in terms of his job. It appears that he needed to meet new people often as well as speak in public when he got out of college, but is this still the case? If his drinking has progressed to the point where he is using alcohol in the morning or throughout the day, does he even have a job, or is it in jeopardy?

Some severe alcoholics can function very well and are able to drink without anyone around them realizing the extent of their use. Thus, Tom's employers and coworkers may or may not realize the extent of his problem. If he continually has to face these difficult social situations, medication may be helpful.

Although, as stated, buspirone does not show significant interaction effects with alcohol (1), Stein et al. (2) point out that this medication also has not been shown to be truly effective in the treatment of social anxiety disorder. It is likely that Tom would find relief from his symptoms of anxiety if he were to use a benzodiazepine, but the abuse potential of this class of drugs and the risk of additive and potentially lethal combination of benzodiazepines and alcohol makes this an inadvisable course of action. Further, the beneficial effect tends to be only temporary.

It is generally recommended that the serotonin reuptake inhibitors (SSRI), especially fluvoxamine, paroxetine and sertraline, are the first-line choice for treatment of panic disorder (2,3). A lack of significant interaction of any of the medications in combination with alcohol makes them particularly useful for this patient (4). At this time, however, given the question of idiosyncratic liver toxicity and nefazodone administration, this medication cannot be recommended for a patient such as Tom, who is at risk of significant liver disease. More information is needed. In addition, insufficient data exist regarding the efficacy of mirtazapine and venlafaxine. Given venlafaxine's hepatic metabolism, it should not be given to Tom if his liver shows any signs of compromise.

Once a medication regimen has been established, Tom is going to face some difficult issues. One will be confronting the vagaries of his job. Is it true that the "three martini lunch" was expected? Or, had he simply volunteered for the clientele who would desire such? Early in his recovery, constant exposure to alcohol and the temptation to use it may be more than he can tolerate. Although offering him disulfiram to act as a deterrent to using or naltrexone to decrease his appetite for alcohol may be helpful, he still needs to be out of the environment where alcohol is in constant use, if possible. He could try transferring to another part of the company with different clientele. If this is not possible, he might try having non-drinking coworkers, colleagues from Alcoholics Anonymous, or his spouse attend luncheons with him. Failing this, he may have to start looking for another job.

CASE 13-2

Elaine, 34 years old, remembered quite well when she first smoked a joint. She was 11 years of age, and her stepfather had given it to her. It was a bribe, the first of many. He would get her high or drunk in exchange for her silence that he was sexually molesting her. That's how the years went for her: you drank or you drugged so you didn't feel. You drank or you drugged so you didn't remember. Drugs became a way of life. When she found cocaine, she found a friend. With cocaine she didn't care what anyone said or did. With cocaine she felt good—as though nothing could hurt her. When she wanted to improve her life, however, and tried to get clean, she found herself reliving the awful times all over again. She saw his face and smelled his rancid tobacco breath. She felt the shame as though it was all new. At times, Elaine would wake up in the night screaming. She actually thought it was happening again, it was so real. She was sure she was going insane. Having a heart attack or smoking herself to death had to be better than reliving the humiliation and pain she had kept submerged in crack for so many years.

Elaine's case brings a dilemma familiar to treatment providers: the woman with posttraumatic stress disorder (PTSD) whose symptoms worsen dramatically as she tries to abstain from substances of abuse. The therapist performs a balancing act with someone such as Elaine that truly tests the clinician's skills: address the flashbacks but do not delve too deeply into the trauma until the patient has some degree of resilience and alternative coping skills as she approaches the issues of trauma. Without having learned any relapse prevention skills, her first reaction will be to revert to using when she begins to confront her past. Acknowledge that flashbacks may become more common and severe as she begins to gain some sobriety. She needs help to deal with the flashbacks but in a relatively nonthreatening fashion.

As with many abused children, Elaine was "bought off" by the perpetrator with alcohol and other drugs, and found them both satisfying and numbing. From a very young age, these became her primary strategies for coping with pain and adversity. During her teens, a time when young people are supposed to be learning more adult strategies for interacting with others and dealing with difficult situations, Elaine was anesthetizing herself from the world. The young age at which she was started on those substances further increased the likelihood she would continue to use and become dependent on them.

Many medications have been used to treat the symptoms of PTSD, including antidepressants, antipsychotics, and benzodiazepines. The lack of efficacy of benzodiazepines, except for the relief of very acute symptoms of distress, their addictive potential, and Elaine's greater risk of abusing such a drug, make this medication an undesirable treatment for her (5,6). Antipsychotic drugs have no place here, because Elaine does not show any signs of psychosis, unless her flashbacks can be interpreted as a psychotic symptom. Regardless of the interpretation, a controlled study by Sernyak et al. (7) failed to show any benefit of such medications in the treatment of PTSD.

Support exists for the use of antidepressants in the treatment of this disorder. As noted in Chapter 11, in regard to the treatment of depression, animal studies have shown that SSRI, other than sertraline, increase seizure activity in conjunction with stimulants (8). Whether this applies to humans is not known. Nevertheless, this medication may be the safest agent to use, as data are lacking regarding the efficacy of nefazodone, mirtazapine, and venlafaxine, although no contraindication now exists to their use (9).

Once medication has been chosen, much work remains to be done for a patient such as Elaine, because a great deal of psychotherapy, rather than pharmacotherapy, must occur.

CASE 13-2A

Elaine has been abstinent for 6 months. She has been comfortable on sertraline (100 mg) during that time; she sleeps well and has returned to work. The feelings of helpless rage she has had for so many years are not so strong now. Further, although her stepfather is dead and she will never be able to confront him about his abuse, she has written him a letter telling him about her hatred and fear. The letter gave her a sense of tremendous freedom and she has been generally more relaxed since writing it. Abruptly, Elaine canceled a session with her addiction counselor and went on a 3-day bender.

Such a relapse is common and, to the inexperienced treatment provider, a frustrating scenario in dealing with the dually diagnosed patient with PTSD. The clinician and patient need to discuss the relapse at length to identify the events leading up to it, who the patient was with, where she went, how much she used, and so on. Possibly, she was "preparing" for a relapse long before it occurred. Patients can set up a relapse by avoiding support meetings, stopping counseling sessions, violating the rules of their relapse prevention plans, and associating with using buddies. It is equally possible, however, that no one, including Elaine, saw the relapse coming. If this is the case, she and her counselor can learn a great deal from it. Was anything different happening in her life before she relapsed? Any new stresses? Sometimes a birthday, the anniversary of a specific event, a death, an accident, or other major occasion can act as a trigger. Did she get back with using friends or go back to old haunts where she used to use?

In Elaine's case, the trigger was one she did not expect. Elaine had always avoided blaming her mother for permitting the abuse to occur. She refused to look at the fact that her mother was always in the house when the abuse occurred and that it would have been extremely difficult for her not to have known what was going on. Immediately before her cocaine binge, Elaine had a sudden memory of seeing her mother in the doorway once when her stepfather was molesting her.

As noted in Chapter 12, flashbacks are powerful relapse cues to substance use. Despite having a number of safeguards in place, Elaine still was not ready for having her denial stripped away so completely and she reverted to an old coping pattern. At this juncture, she can go either way. She may be able to come back from the brief binge to work on her sobriety and her issues simultaneously, having developed skills for dealing with both. On the other hand, she may find that the pain is too great for her right now and revert to cocaine anesthesia for awhile. Regardless of which way she eventually goes, her next round of therapy will be on firmer ground with a greater awareness of the issues.

CASE 13-3

Tracy, 29, had her first full-blown anxiety attack while smoking a joint with friends. She noticed she had started becoming increasingly paranoid when she smoked, but had laughed it off to "bad dope." Then one night, she found herself watching people's hands as they came out of the kitchen—convinced they would be bringing knives with them for . . . some reason. She couldn't exactly say what. That was the night it happened. A man came out of the kitchen and raised his hands to his waist, the way she had seen knife fights in the movies. Her heart rate, already increased from the marijuana, just took off, beating faster and faster. She knew he meant her harm. It became difficult to breathe. She was already fuzzy from the dope, but she thought she would faint. She sat with her head down until the world stopped spinning and her heart slowed down. She tried marijuana a few more times, but each time the same thing happened. Things got so bad that just thinking about getting high was enough to make her heart race and the world to feel as though it was closing in on her. Once her heart stopped racing, she found a strong swig of whiskey that was passed to her actually made things better. Within moments, inexperienced as she was with alcohol, the warmth flowed through her and she quickly felt better.

Tracy is a good example of both anticipatory anxiety and cannabis-induced anxiety. Although for many individuals, both with and without anxiety disorders, cannabis has a calming and relaxing effect, a significant percentage of those with anxiety disorders will note marked worsening of this condition when they use this drug. In addition, numerous case examples exist of persons who experience their first ever panic attacks while under the influence of cannabis. Marijuana use by such individuals tends to be self-limited because it is so uncomfortable and the anticipatory component is so great.

The problem, however, is that although patients such as Tracy may stop using marijuana, it does not mean the panic attacks will stop. Further, she discovered something that many others like her have found: alcohol makes things better, thus strongly reinforcing its use (10–13).

Because Tracy knows that she can have instant relief from her distress by using alcohol, it will be difficult to engage her in treatment. Further, of the medications that have been shown to be of short-term benefit in treating panic disorder, tricyclic antidepressants (TCA), SSRI, and benzodiazepines, only the latter show rapid symptoms relief. As long as she is drinking, has no skills at abstinence, and is looking for a quick fix, Tracy is not a good candidate for this class of drugs. In fact, many treatment providers in the addictions field would argue that she would never be a good candidate for such an intervention regardless of the skills she possessed or the amount of clean time she has had because of the abuse potential of the benzodiazepines.

Not yet described is her drinking pattern (i.e., daily, episodically, only when she feels panicky, all through the day). Thus, additional information is needed. Does she show evidence of physiologic dependence (e.g., withdrawal symptoms)? Will she require help with detoxification? Regardless of the answers to these questions, once she is detoxified, if this is indicated, she will need something to help her through the very frightening experience of panic attacks. It is probably safest to start a patient such as Tracy on an SSRI. Even if she continues to drink, she will likely experience some symptom relief with one of these medications while efforts are made to engage her in treatment and help her to achieve some sobriety. The potential for severe or even lethal interaction if alcohol is mixed with either the TCA or a benzodiazepine makes using either of these a poor choice for the individual who is actively drinking.

While Tracy is developing a social milieu that is supportive of her sobriety, she can be learning various relaxation and breathing techniques to help her through the most frightening episodes. It would not be unusual for a patient such as Tracy to have a difficult time initiating any degree of abstinence early on. She is afraid of being afraid. She has found an effective remedy for the misery she experiences when she has a panic attack, and it will be difficult for her to have the courage not to use it. For her, combining relaxation techniques and medication may be essential to get her through the first frightening weeks of trying to slow down and eventually stop her drinking.

REFERENCES

1. Rush CR, Griffitchs RR. Acute participant-rated and behavioral effects of alprazolam and buspirone, alone and in combination with ethanol, in normal volunteers. *Exp Clin Psychopharmacol* 1997; 5(1):28–36.
2. Stein DJ, Westenberg HGM, Liebowitz MR. Social anxiety disorder and generalized anxiety disorder: serotonergic and dopaminergic neurocircuitry. *J Clin Psychiatry* 2002;63(Suppl 6):12–19.
3. Nunes EV, McGrath PJ, Quitkin FM. Treating anxiety in patients with alcoholism. *J Clin Psychiatry* 1995;56(Suppl 2):3–9.
4. Van Harten J, Stevens LA, Baghoebar M, et al. Fluvoxamine does not interact with alcohol or potentiate alcohol related impairment of cognitive function. *Clin Pharmacol Ther* 1992;52:427–435.
5. Braun P, Greenberg D, Dasberg H, et al. Core symptoms of posttraumatic stress disorder unimproved by alprazolam treatment. *J Clin Psychiatry* 1990;51:226–238.
6. Gelpin E, Bonne O, Peri T, et al. Treatment of recent trauma survivors with benzodiazepines: a prospective study. *J Clin Psychiatry* 1996;57:390–394.
7. Sernyak MJ, Kosten TR, Fontana A, et al. Neuroleptic use in the treatment of post-traumatic stress disorder. *Psychiatric Q* 2001; 72(3):197–213.
8. O'Dell LE, George FR, Ritz MC. Antidepressant drugs appear to enhance cocaine induced toxicity. *Exp Clin Psychopharmacol* 2000; 8(1):133–141.
9. Davidson JRT. Recognition and treatment of posttraumatic stress disorder. *JAMA* 2001;286(5):584–588.
10. George DT, Lindquist T, Ragan PW, et al. Effect of alcoholism on the incidence of lactate induced panic attacks. *Biol Psychiatry* 1997;42(11):992–999.
11. Marshall JR. Alcohol and substance abuse in panic disorder. *J Clin Psychiatry* 1997;58(Suppl 2):46–49.
12. Kushner MG, Mackenzie TB, Fiszdon J, et al. The effects of alcohol consumption on laboratory induced panic and state anxiety. *Arch Gen Psychiatry* 1996;53(3):264–270.
13. Lepola U. Alcohol and depression in panic disorder. *Acta Psychiatr Scand Suppl* 1994;377:33–35.

Special Populations Among the Dually Diagnosed: Women and the Elderly

1. The elderly
   a. Little concrete data exist regarding this population and substance misuse
   b. Current middle-aged Americans have very different substance use history than the current elderly
   c. Body handles alcohol differently with age
      i. Not a difference with hepatic metabolism
      ii. Issue is of volume of distribution
      iii. Same dose of alcohol will result in higher dose in individual at 60 years of age than it did at 35 years of age
      iv. Cirrhosis fatal 7% of time in those younger than 50 years of age; 50% of time in those more than 60 years of age
      v. "Benefits" of alcohol are highly variable
         (a) Differ between sexes, between individuals
         (b) Differ also according to amount consumed
   d. Prescription drug abuse common in the elderly
      i. Elderly use a great number of prescriptions
      ii. Elderly are among the least compliant with medications
      iii. Narcotic analgesic and benzodiazepine misuse are common
      iv. Body also handles nonabusable drugs (e.g., lithium and valproic acid) differently
2. Women
   a. Some issues regarding dual diagnoses are unique when dealing with women
   b. Substance use disorders less often diagnosed in women
   c. Once diagnosed, fewer treatment options
      i. Less likely to be referred for treatment
      ii. Less likely to be supported by family or significant others to seek treatment
   d. Women face a number of barriers to treatment
      i. Childcare
      ii. Transportation
      iii. Fear of losing custody if their substance use is made known
   e. Women with both psychiatric and substance use disorders may experience perimenstrual changes in their disorders
   f. Pregnancy may not be recognized by the woman until well into the second trimester because of a variety of factors
      i. Makes good prenatal care more difficult
      ii. Women may avoid both prenatal care and treatment for substance use disorders, fearing legal entanglements or that the infant will be removed
   g. Menopause affects and is affected by both substance use and psychiatric disorders
      i. Symptoms of schizophrenia and bipolar disorder can worsen at this time
      ii. Depression, in general, can be harder to treat because of the intensity of hormone fluctuation
      iii. Alcohol-dependent women experience menopause earlier than those who are not; such women are at higher risk of cardiovascular problems and osteoporosis

INTRODUCTION

Previous chapters have included case examples of individuals from populations that present special or unique challenges for the treatment provider. An elderly depressed alcohol-dependent man poses more health and suicide risks than a younger counterpart. A woman with bipolar disorder and episodic cocaine use may present with cyclical changes in either disorder that are associated with her menstrual cycle. A pregnant woman with schizophrenia and cocaine use poses legal, obstetric, and psychiatric problems for the treatment team. This chapter focuses on these populations—the elderly and women—to stress some of the issues that are of particular concern to the clinician treating the dually diagnosed.

THE ELDERLY

It has become cliché to point out that the population in the United States is aging. More people are living to retirement age and beyond than ever before. Little research in the past, however, focused on substance misuse by the elderly. Thus, little is known about what to expect in terms of substance misuse and the older generation. It is known that men and women tend to decrease their alcohol use after the age of 60 years and that the elderly, traditionally, have used fewer illicit drugs than have younger persons (1). The current generation in its middle years, especially women, has a substantially different substance use history than the current elderly. It is likely that as this group ages findings regarding their substance use will change dramatically (2).

How the body handles alcohol changes with age. Although liver metabolism does not change, blood levels do because of a change in the body's distribution of lean muscle mass to water. Thus, individuals, at 60 years of age, will experience a higher blood alcohol level for a given amount of alcohol than they did at 30 (1). That alcohol has positive cardiac and cognitive benefits has been widely heralded. The fact that this is highly individualized, dose-related, and differs between the sexes has not received as much attention (3). Further, men and women experience substance use-related physical and mental difficulties at a different rate and over a different time course. Alcohol, for example, causes cirrhosis and cognitive damage in women after a lower level of consumption and after a briefer period of exposure than it does in men. In addition, although the mortality rate of cirrhosis is only 7% in a person under 50 years of age, it is more than 50% in someone over the age of 60, making a "safe" level of usage extremely important.

Prescription drug misuse is a particular problem among the older population. Persons more than 65 years of age account for 14% of the population but use nearly a third of all prescriptions (4). Further, this group tends to be noncompliant with its medications. It is estimated that half to three quarters of all medications prescribed for the elderly are taken incorrectly, with the chances of noncompliance increasing with the number of drugs the individual takes (4). In fact, according to the National Institute on Drug Abuse, older Americans are the least compliant with medications of all population groups (5).

Iatrogenic dependence on narcotic pain relievers poses a significant problem in this population because of the risk of falls and fractures as well as adverse effects on cognition. Benzodiazepine use also increases with age and the elderly tend to be on relatively high doses, posing risks similar to narcotics (1). Further, for individuals with mild dementia, forgetting whether or not they have taken their medication and accidentally overdosing is not a trivial issue.

Medication problems in the elderly come not just from misuse of, or dependence on, addictive medications. Such also arise as a result of changes in how the body responds to nondependent-inducing drugs. As the individual ages, the body begins to handle drugs differently. The mood stabilizers, lithium and valproic acid, for example, take twice as long to clear the body on average in an individual above 65 years of age as in a 30-year-old (6). In the person using other substances as well, this can pose an even greater danger.

CASE 14-1

Jim L., a retired accountant 71 years of age, was brought to the clinic one June morning for his increasingly erratic behavior. His daughter and her husband, who lived close by, indicated that in the preceding few weeks he had begun calling them at odd hours of the night ranting about news events, past slights, and future plans. He appeared to be sleeping little and spending a lot of money on equipment for an "invention" he claimed would make them all wealthy. Further, it appeared he was drinking more than usual. They had never known him to have a drinking problem, but lately when he called, his speech seemed slurred. They had seen this behavior a number of years before when he had been hospitalized for mania, although they were not aware of any recurrence. Jim refused hospitalization, but indicated he knew from past experience that he had a "lithium deficiency," for which he would take replacement therapy. Five weeks after initiation of lithium treatment Jim was brought to the hospital by his family. His speech was unintelligible, his gait was quite unsteady. A very coarse tremor could be seen in both his arms and upper body. Jim's lithium level was found to be 2.1 and a nurse noted a strong odor of alcohol on his breath, although no alcohol level was obtained.

A number of things needed to be known once the crisis of Jim's lithium toxicity is past. One, of course, is did he intentionally try to kill himself? Jim has several risk factors for suicide: he is widowed, a male with a prior and recent history of affective disorder, and, apparently, has been drinking But how much?

Jim was a daily drinker for many years, coming home to two or three mixed drinks per evening. By definition, this made him a heavy drinker, although it never interfered with his job, social life, or health. Now living alone and retired, he has time on his hands. He may or may not be drinking more. Regardless, three mixed drinks is a substantial amount of alcohol if it is mixed in a

Table 14-1.   Age-related issues

Alcohol	Higher level at a given dose because of volume of distribution
Lithium	Reduced clearance with age (increased level/dose)
Medication compliance	Increased risk of noncompliance with age and with comorbidity in general
Psychiatric	Increased risk of suicide because of gender, age, loss (wife), substance use, and affective disorder

bar, where the business wants to see to it that each drink does not exceed the 1.5 ounces—what a "drink" is supposed to measure. It is impossible to guess how much alcohol Jim is actually consuming at home, where people frequently do not measure the alcohol into a glass, but simply pour it.

Jim's body now distributes alcohol differently than it once did. Alcohol *per se* has a dehydrating effect on the body. In addition, at his age the three drinks he consumed 10 years ago now would be expected to produce a higher blood level than it did then. As noted, lithium clearance decreases with age. It turns out Jim knew what his previous dose had been and was not impressed by the much smaller dose his physician had prescribed. Therefore, he had increased it on his own to the dose he had taken many years before. In addition, it is summertime. The combination of decreased lithium clearance, dehydrating effect of hot weather, alcohol, and the aging body's altered handling of alcohol put him in his current situation.

The grandiosity of hypomania or mania always has the potential to significantly impair the patient's judgment. In Jim's case, because of factors related to age and poor choices, things that he might have easily gotten away with in his 30s might have proved fatal in his 70s (Table 14-1).

CASE 14-2

Mrs. H., 73 years of age, had been expected to remain in the hospital only overnight. An adverse reaction to the dye used in a procedure, however, made it necessary to keep her an extra day and night for observation. By the afternoon of the second day she began to complain of generalized discomfort. She stated she had numbness and tingling around her mouth and a feeling that she "wasn't there" or that "things weren't real." Shortly thereafter, she became mute and rigid. A fine diffuse tremor and profuse sweating were noted. The patient did not follow directions nor did she answer questions. Her temperature was slightly elevated, as were her blood pressure and pulse.

Mrs. H. was not known to be taking any medications routinely, although had been prescribed lorazepam on an "as needed basis," per records reviewed by her family physician. Since the death of her husband 2 years before Mrs. H. had been known to suffer from occasional panic attacks and had responded well to periodic benzodiazepine therapy.

It would not be surprising to find that Mrs. H. has been using the "as needed" lorazepam routinely and possibly even in excess of the prescribed doses, which could account for the current symptoms. Reports of catatonia and seizure activity as a result of abrupt withdrawal from benzodiazepines, especially among the elderly, can be found in the literature (7,8). Mrs. H. is of a generation that was frequently prescribed sedatives and hypnotics beginning in their 30s and 40s, at a time when little attention was paid to the potential for physical dependence to such agents to occur.

A review of pharmacy records revealed that Mrs. H. was indeed taking lorazepam routinely, and that two different physicians—her family physician and a cardiac specialist—were prescribing it. An injection of lorazepam was sufficient to restore Mrs. H. completely to her usual mental state.

Such situations can arise innocently enough, although clinicians often jump to the conclusion that they have been "had" and become angry with the patient. The prescriptions may have been obtained under different names (e.g., generic and brand name) and from different pharmacies. The elderly are highly sensitive to the cognitive effects of the benzodiazepines and Mrs. H. may not have been aware of just how much medication she was taking. Because she was told to take the medications "as needed for anxiety," and she felt anxious all the time, she likely felt justified in taking it at every opportunity.

Now, the question is, what to do about the problem? Once patients realize they are unable to discontinue the medication without help, which to them means they are "addicted" to a drug, they are often embarrassed. After all, it is not socially acceptable to be an "addict," and certainly not ladylike, to Mrs. H. She may need a lot of hand-holding to successfully get through a period of detoxification and possible rebound anxiety.

On the other hand, she may actively resist the idea of being weaned from the benzodiazepines despite compelling arguments about the risk of falls and fractures and cognitive difficulties associated with such medications in the elderly. It does appear that Mrs. H. should not be on benzodiazepines. As noted in Chapter 12, this is not the treatment of choice for a condition such as she has, in addition to which she has demonstrated, for whatever reason, she does not use them responsibly.

Mrs. H. should be detoxified from her lorazepam and, if treatment for her anxiety is needed, placed on an SSRI instead. Detoxification can be accomplished in one of several ways. It should be noted, however, benzodiazepine detoxification, in general, has a low success rate—more so among the elderly (9,10), who tend to resist this change.

The detoxification regimen most acceptable to patients but with the lowest overall success rate is to place them on divided doses of the substance on which they are dependent, and to decrease the medication over time. For example, an individual taking 1 mg alprazolam three times per day, could be placed on 0.75 mg three times a day, then 0.5 mg three times per day, and so forth. However, the reason patients feel most positive about this approach is that they are using something familiar, and are also more likely to sabotage the process by taking more than prescribed. Unless the physician prescribes only a day or two of the medication at a time, it then becomes a struggle of wills between the physician and the patient, with the latter demanding more and the former refusing. Plus, when the physician is worried about the possible emergence of seizure activity, it is difficult to refuse to refill a prescription if the patient runs out too soon.

A second approach is to place the patient on a long-acting agent (e.g., clonazepam) twice daily, making sure the patient is stable on this regimen and then gradually decreasing each dose (11). Because the medication is unfamiliar, patients tend to be less accepting of such an approach, although it is the most widely used by practitioners and has a better success rate.

Finally, an approach that has proved safe and effective but is generally resisted by patients is that of hospitalization, abrupt cessation of the benzodiazepine, and initiation of carbamazepine (12). Because this approach has been used on elderly patients, hospitalization is recommended in the event that some unforeseen problem should arise. Despite this approach being safe for detoxification, follow-up shows that most patients revert to benzodiazepine use.

A long-term relationship, reassurance, and firmness are typically necessary to successfully bring a patient such as Mrs. H. through this period.

WOMEN

Treating women with substance use disorders, comorbid or not, presents some special considerations regarding treatment options, barriers to treatment, relapse issues, physical problems, and, of course, pregnancy and menopause. Increasingly, women (particularly older women) are being identified as problem drinkers, where previously this was not the case. Clinicians have generally been less inclined to ask women about substance use. As it is becoming more widely recognized that women do have substance use disorders, increasingly the problem arises of what to do with the woman with a substance use disorder once it has been identified.

Substance misuse is still more likely to be missed among women than among men and, when it is recognized, women are less likely to be recommended for treatment by healthcare providers and by the courts than are their male counterparts. Women are less often referred for treatment by employee assistance programs than are men (13,14). Women tend to encourage partners and other family members to receive treatment for substance abuse disorders. Families and partners of substance-abusing women, on the other hand, are much more likely to deny the existence of such a problem in a female member, which helps her avoid addressing the issue. Thus, pathways by which men have traditionally entered treatment for substance misuse are either unavailable or inconsistently so, to women (15,16).

Once treatment for substance misuse is considered, women face significant barriers to receiving it. First, fewer treatment facilities are available for women, in general. If a woman is pregnant, many programs will reject her because they cannot handle pregnancy-related issues. Women are more likely to have partners who are not supportive of, or are actively resistant to, her entering treatment. Women with substance use disorders often avoid treatment out of fear of rejection, shame, and the belief that they, as women with substance problems, are less socially acceptable than are their male counterparts (16,17).

Women head two thirds of families with children under the age of 18. Fear that admitting to, and receiving help for, a substance misuse problem will cause them to lose custody of their children is another reason women avoid entering addiction treatment. Also, wondering who will care for minor children while she is in treatment for her substance use problem is a major issue that may deter her from receiving help. Further, transportation to and from treatment, especially if the woman has small children, can pose a major problem for women with substance use disorders (18–20).

Pregnancy and the dramatic hormonal changes that punctuate the female reproductive life can have a significant influence on both psychiatric and substance use disorders. For example, a strong suggestion is that women may be less sensitive to the effects of cocaine during some phases of the menstrual cycle and, thus, may be at higher risk of abusing large quantities of cocaine to overcome this fact. Substance-misusing women often experience premenstrual craving for, and then use, substances. They may be particularly at risk for relapse to substance use at these times (21–23). Some question also arises to whether some women with schizophrenia and bipolar disorder may experience perimenstrual exacerbation of their symptoms, although not all women with these diagnoses experience such (24–27).

The pregnant substance user presents the clinician with a whole different set of problems. More than 19% of pregnant women surveyed in 1992 admitted to using just alcohol during their pregnancy (28). It is not at all uncommon for pregnant women who misuse substances to be unaware they are pregnant until they feel the fetus move. This happens for a variety of reasons. Women on stimulants can lose much body fat and be unable to sustain regular ovulation and menstruation, making it difficult for them to track their natural cycle. Generally, erratic lifestyle and debility of the chronic alcoholic or other type of drug user can also contribute to such. Further, the woman may simply be so tied up in her drug use that she is oblivious to whatever else is going on about her. If she is also psychotic, this can further contribute to her lack of awareness, for example, of pregnancy.

It is often difficult to accurately gauge gestational age because of the factors listed above, in addition to the fact that drug-exposed pregnancies tend not to be healthy ones. Babies born to substance-abusing women tend to be small at birth, regardless of gestational age (i.e., premature or not), because of the mother's poor weight gain and lack of prenatal care. Many pregnant women with substance use disorders want to seek help for their problem and to obtain prenatal care in order to improve the outcome of their pregnancies. Such women often avoid both, however, out of fear of punishment for their substance use or that their infants will be taken away from them at birth if they make their substance use known.

Menopause and the perimenopausal period is influenced by and, in turn, influences both substance use and major psychiatric disorders. Women with alcohol dependence, for example, experience an earlier onset of menopause (29). In the postmenopausal period, they show markedly different hormonal levels than their nonalcoholic female counterparts and are more likely to develop osteoporosis. Further, evidence indicates that psychotic symptoms can worsen among women with schizophrenia during the perimenopausal time (30). Likewise, women with bipolar disorder not being treated with hormone replacement are more likely to experience affective lability (31). Estrogen, in general, appears to have an antidepressant effect in postmenopausal women with mood disorders and its lack or insufficiency can make the treatment of affective problems difficult (32,33).

Although comorbidity is common, it is definitely the rule rather than the exception it comes to women with substance use disorders. Up to 75% of women in treatment for alcohol and other drug problems have been victims of incest or other sexual abuse. Such women fear that confronting the addiction issue will cause painful and unresolved issues to reemerge. Women with substance use disorders have four times the incidence of unipolar depression as men and three times that of non–substance-abusing women. Likewise, such women experience panic disorders three and a half times more often than similarly diagnosed men and their depression and anxiety disorders appear to predate the onset of substance misuse 60% of the time. Women with mania and schizophrenia may be slightly more likely than men with these disorders to be concomitantly diagnosed as having alcohol or other drug problems, although such problems are common in men as well (16,34–36). Women with substance use disorders generally have a rate of completed suicide that is 18 to 21 times that of a nonsubstance abuser, or about three times as high as male substance abusers. The rate for women with dual diagnoses is even higher (37–41).

Women with alcohol problems tend to have partners with the same, whereas men may or may not. Thus, if a woman attempts to get treatment for her substance use disorder and her partner does not, either she will need to terminate the relationship or she will be unlikely to improve her substance use.

CASE 14-3

Mrs. S., 49 years of age, is slender and active. She presented to her family physician with complaints of fatigue and sleep disturbance. On physical examination, her blood pressure was 138/98. During conversation, she became tearful and expressed concern that her husband was likely to lose his job because of absenteeism related to his drinking. She indicated that she

*often called in to cover for him, but that the excuses were no
longer being accepted. Further, Mrs. S. indicated she too was
missing work because of the need to stay home to care for her
husband.*

A number of issues need to be addressed further in this case,
and many questions asked. The patient is 49 years of age, "slender and active." Why then is she hypertensive? In addition, she
has presented with symptoms highly suggestive of depression.
More questions in this regard should be asked, especially about
hopelessness and suicidal thoughts. Further, increased substance use and concomitant domestic instability increase the
risk of violence. Have there been any episodes of hostility? Has
Mrs. S. been physically abused or is she afraid of her husband?
Finally, is Mrs. S. drinking as well? Is this contributing to her
own absenteeism?

Hypertension has long been known to be associated with alcohol use, although most early studies looked only at men (42,43).
Recent research has suggested that elevated diastolic blood pressure, with normal or near normal systolic blood pressure, is a
common finding among women with alcohol use disorders and
may be an early marker for this problem in women (44). Knowing
this, the clinician should be alerted to the very real likelihood that
Mrs. S. too has a drinking problem.

When directly confronted about this issue, Mrs. S. tearfully admitted that she found herself drinking more in the evenings when
she was home. She felt lonely and frustrated, even though her
husband was home. He was emotionally absent and often physically ill from his drinking. She felt resentful at having to care for
him and angry at the fact that his drinking had taken such a toll
on their lives and their finances. Although not admitting to being
alcohol dependent, Mrs. S. did admit that she needed to drink less
than was currently the case.

Regardless of whether or not Mrs. S.'s husband seeks help for his
drinking problem, the patient should be encouraged to seek help
for her own. She cannot wait for him to stop drinking to address
her own difficulties. It is true that their relationship will be considerably strained if she succeeds in drying out and he continues to
drink. It is also true that such a scenario will act as a considerable
threat to her future abstinence if the couple stays together. Nevertheless, she is the designated patient, and her drinking is seriously
affecting her health and her occupational functioning. The principal concern here is Mrs. S.

At her age, Mrs. S. is likely experiencing symptoms of the
menopause. Depending on how long and how much she has used
alcohol, these symptoms may be more advanced than for other
women of her age. Information about her menstrual history
should be obtained. How heavily is she bleeding? Are her periods
regular? If it is determined that she is depressed, is there a cyclical change in her depression? Chapter 10 emphasized that simultaneous treatment of depression and alcohol dependence is
desirable. Although Mrs. S. should be considered for antidepressant medication, she should also be referred for a physical examination and consideration for hormonal regulation depending

Table 14-2.   Female-related issues

Diagnosis and treatment
Identified less often as having substance use disorders
Referred for treatment less often
Fewer treatment options available

Barriers to treatment
Childcare
Transportation
Fear of losing custody if admitting to problem
Nonsupportive family or significant other

Physical differences
Higher blood level at same dose of alcohol
Perimenstrual changes in tolerance/reaction to some substances
Negative physical effects at lower doses after shorter time of exposure
Menopause modified by or modifies both psychiatric and substance
    use disorders

Psychiatric
May or may not experience perimenstrual exacerbation
Perimenopausal exacerbation of symptoms common
Psychopathology more common in females with substance use disorders

on what is obtained in the history, physical examination, and laboratory screening. As noted, estrogen alone can have significant antidepressant effects (Table 14-2).

REFERENCES

1. Fingerhood M. Substance abuse in older people. *J Am Geriatr Soc* 2000;48(8):985–995.
2. Szwabo PA. Substance abuse in the older woman. *Clin Geriatr Med* 1993;9(1):197–209.
3. Zuccola G, Orider G, Pedone C, et al. Dose related impact of alcohol consumption on cognitive function in advanced age. Results of a multicenter survey. *Alcohol Clin Exp Res* 2001;25(12):1743–1748.
4. Avorn J. Drug prescribing, drug taking, adverse reactions and compliance in elderly patients. In: Salzman C, ed. *Clinical geriatric psychopharmacology*. Baltimore: Williams & Wilkins, 1998:21–50.
5. Abuse NIoD. *Prescription drugs: abuse and addiction*. Bethesda, MD: National Institutes of Health, 2001.
6. von Moltke LL, Abernethy DR, Greenblatt DJ. Kinetics and dynamics of psychotropic drugs in the elderly. In: Salzman C, ed. *Clinical geriatric psychopharmacology*. Baltimore: Williams & Wilkins, 1998:70–96.
7. Rosebush PI, Mazurek MF. Catatonia after benzodiazepine withdrawal. *J Clin Psychopharmacol* 1996;16(4):315–319.
8. Deuschle M, Lederbogen F. Benzodiazepine withdrawal-induced catatonia. *Pharmacopsychiatry* 2001;34(1):41–42.
9. Schweizer E, Rickels K, Case W, et al. Long-term therapeutic use of benzodiazepines II. Effect of gradual taper. *Arch Gen Psychiatry* 1990;47:708–715.

10. Schweizer E, Rickels K. Benzodiazepine dependence and with-drawal: a review of the syndrome and its clinical management. *Acta Psychiatr Scand Suppl* 1998;98(393):95–101.

11. Rickels K, DeMartinis N, Rynn M, et al. Pharmacologic strategies for discontinuing benzodiazepine treatment. *J Clin Psychopharmacol* 1999;19(Suppl 6):12s–16s.

12. Schweizer E, Rickels K, Case W, et al. Carbamazepine treatment in patients discontinuing long term benzodiazepine therapy: effects on withdrawal severity and outcome. *Arch Gen Psychiatry* 1991;48(5):448–452.

13. Treatment CfSA. *Practical approaches in the treatment of women who abuse alcohol and other drugs.* Rockville, MD: Department of Health and Human Services, 1995.

14. Smith L. Help seeking in alcohol dependent females. *Alcohol Alcohol* 1992;27(1):3–9.

15. O'Connor LE, Inaba D, Weiss J, et al. Shame, guilt, and depression in men and women in recovery from addiction. *J Subst Abuse Treat* 1994;11(6):503–510.

16. Blume S. Sexuality and stigma: the alcoholic woman. *Alcohol Health and Research World* 1991;15(2):139–146.

17. Blumenthal SJ. Women and substance abuse: a new national focus. In: Wetherington CL, Roman AB, eds. *Drug addiction research and the health of women.* Rockville, MD, National Institute on Drug Abuse, 1998:13–32.

18. Coletti SD. Service providers and treatment access issues. In: Wetherington CL, Roman AB, eds. *Drug addiction research and the health of women.* Rockville, MD, National Institute on Drug Abuse, 1998.

19. Wilsnack SC. Patterns and trends in women's drinking: recent findings and some implications for prevention. In: Howard JM, Martin SE, Mail PD, et al. *Women and alcohol: issues for prevention and research,* Vol Research Monograph No. 32. Bethesda, MD: National Institutes of Health, 1996.

20. Commerce USDo. *Statistical abstract of the United States, 1992.* Washington, DC: US Government Printing Office, 1993.

21. Bowersox JA. Cocaine affects men and women differently, NIDA study shows. *NIDA Notes* 1996;January/February.

22. Randall CLR, James S, DelBoca FK, et al. Telescoping of landmark events associated with drinking: a gender comparison. *J Stud Alcohol* 1999;(March):252–260.

23. Allen SS, Hatsukami D, Christianson D, et al. Symptomatology and energy intake during the menstrual cycle in smoking women. *J Subst Abuse* 1996;8(3):303–319.

24. Magharious WG, Donald C, Amico E. Relationship of gender and menstrual status to symptoms and medication side effects in patients with schizophrenia. *Psychiatry Res* 1998;77(3):159–166.

25. Harris AH. Menstrually related symptom changes in women with schizophrenia. *Schizophr Res* 1997;27(1):93–99.

26. Leibenluft E, Ashman SB, Feldman-Naim S, et al. Lack of relationship between menstrual cycle phase and mood in a sample of women with rapid cycling bipolar disorder. *Biol Psychiatry* 1999; 46(4):577–580.

27. Hallonquist JD, Seeman MV, Lang M, et al. Variation in symptom severity over the menstrual cycle of schizophrenia. *Biol Psychiatry* 1993;33(3):207–209.

28. *National pregnancy and health survey: drug use among women delivering live births in 1992*. Rockville, MD: National Institutes on Drug Abuse, 1996.
29. Torgerson DJ, Campbell MK, Thomas RE, et al. Alcohol consumption may influence onset of menopause. *BMJ* 1997;315(7101):188.
30. Seeman MV. Does menopause intensify symptoms in schizophrenia? In: Lewis-Hall F, Williams TS, eds. *Psychiatric illness in women: emerging treatment and research*. Washington, DC: American Psychiatric Press, 2002:239–248.
31. Freeman MP, Smith KW, Freeman SA, et al. The impact of reproductive events on the course of bipolar disorder in women. *J Clin Psychiatry* 2002;63(4):284–287.
32. Rasgon NL, Altshuler LL, Fairbanks LA, et al. Estrogen replacement therapy in the treatment of major depressive disorder in perimenopausal women. *J Clin Psychiatry* 2002;63(Suppl 7):45–48.
33. Soares CdN, Almeida OP, Joffe H, et al. Efficacy of estradiol for the treatment of depressive disorders in perimenopausal women: a double-blind, randomized, placebo-controlled trial. *Arch Gen Psychiatry* 2001;58(6):529–534.
34. Regier DA, Farmer ME, Rae DS, et al. Comorbidity of mental disorders with alcohol and other drug abuse: results from the Epidemiological Catchment Area study. *JAMA* 1990;264(19):2511–2518.
35. Kandel DB, Warner LA, Kessler RC. The epidemiology of substance use and dependence among women. In: Wetherington CL, Roman AB, eds. *Drug addiction research and the health of women*. Rockville, MD: National Institutes on Drug Abuse, 1998.
36. Merikangas KR, Stevens DE. Substance abuse among women: familial factors and comorbidity. In: Wetherington CL, Roman AB, eds. *Drug addiction research and the health of women*. Rockville, MD: National Institutes on Drug Abuse, 1998.
37. Eronen M, Hakola P, Tiihonen J. Mental disorders and homicidal behavior in Finland. *Arch Gen Psychiatry* 1996;53(6):497–501.
38. Roizen J. Issues in the epidemiology of alcohol and violence. In: Martin SE, ed. *Alcohol and interpersonal violence: fostering multidisciplinary perspectives*, Vol. 93-3496. Rockville, MD: National Institutes of Health, 1993.
39. Scott J, Johnson S, Menezes P, et al. Substance misuse and risk of aggression and offending among the severely mentally ill. *Br J Psychiatry* 1998;172(4):345–350.
40. Hodgins S, Mednick SA, Brennan PA, et al. Mental disorder and crime: evidence from a Danish birth cohort. *Arch Gen Psychiatry* 1996;53(6):489–496.
41. Harris EC, Barraclough B. Excess mortality of mental disorder. *Br J Psychiatry* 1998;173(7):11–53.
42. Moreira LB, Fuchs FD, Moraes RS, et al. Alcohol intake and blood pressure: the importance of time elapsed since last drink. *J Hypertens* 1998;16(2):175–180.
43. York JL, Hirsch JA. Association between blood pressure and lifetime drinking patterns in moderate drinkers. *J Stud Alcohol* 1997;58(5):480–485.
44. Seppa K, Laippala P, Sillanaukee P. High diastolic blood pressure: common among women who are heavy drinkers. *Alcohol Clin Exp Res* 1996;20(1):47–51.

15

Other Drugs of Abuse and Mental Illness

1. Drugs other than those discussed are also used in various areas
   a. Substance use varies by region, culture, and socioeconomic strata
   b. MDMA (3,4-methylenedioxymethamphetamine), methamphetamine, others are around
2. Phencyclidine (PCP) is again popular in some places
   a. Now used only as an animal tranquilizer
   b. Can produce a psychosis identical to schizophrenia
   c. Users can hurt others without feeling pain because they are using an anesthetic
   d. Treatment of the user
      i. Memory deficits are a long lasting, but not permanent problem
      ii. Detoxification is not necessary
      iii. Acidification of the urine is helpful but can be difficult to achieve
      iv. No evidence that sedation or antipsychotics reduce the time course of psychosis
   e. Effect on newborn: unknown
   f. Depression in PCP may be protracted: serotonin reuptake inhibitors (SSRI) may be helpful
3. Polysubstance misuse with heavy emphasis on amphetamines and MDMA
   a. Both drugs can cause long-term or permanent central nervous system damage
   b. Both affect serotonin system
   c. Depression immediately following use of either is common
      i. Because of serotonin effect of drugs, SSRI may be helpful
      ii. Depression can be difficult to treat
4. Polysubstance misuse, beginning with inhalants, can produce a mixed picture
   a. Inhalant can cause permanent abnormal movements from brain damage
   b. Substance-induced psychosis is typically short lived, although can be protracted
      i. Anecdotal reports support use of typical antipsychotics for treatment: good data lacking
      ii. Anecdotal reports support atypical antipsychotics: good data lacking
   c. Depression not uncommon in wake of inhalant misuse

Substances, other than those discussed in other chapters, are used by various groups in the United States, with strong regional, cultural, and socioeconomic differences seen. "Ecstasy" (MDMA) is used by middle-class, young adults. "Ice" (smokeable amphetamine) is available on the coasts and in Hawaii, and appears sporadically in rural areas. "Cat" (methcathinone) is a particularly "dirty drug" whose extraction leaves much particulate matter behind in the product, including bits of battery acid, and is used primarily in the Midwest. γ-hydroxybutyrate (GHB) has a strong following on the West Coast and into Colorado. Each of these substances, as with all other drugs of abuse, can cause serious psychiatric effects of their own or worsen preexisting psychiatric conditions. Cases presented below are composites of patients who have used such drugs.

One drug whose popularity has waxed and waned over the years but that appears to be on the rise again in some parts of the United States is that of phencyclidine (PCP). Developed initially as a human anesthetic, problems quickly emerged among individuals treated with this medication including hallucinations, disorientation, and combativeness that resulted in its being discontinued for human use. PCP is now used only in veterinary medicine in the United States.

PCP can be taken orally or smoked. A popular mode of administration is to combine it with marijuana and smoke the two together. The user may experience visual hallucinations, synesthesias and altered bodily sensations. Some particularly sensitive users can exhibit a psychotic process identical to schizophrenia that can last for an extended period of time.

Users of PCP have a reputation for being unpredictable and potentially dangerous. At one time a strong belief was that individuals who used PCP were more dangerous than users of other substances of abuse. It is not entirely clear that this is the case, as aggregate data show that individuals who perpetrated violent acts and tested positive for PCP also tested positive for other substances (1,2). What is clear is that PCP is an anesthetic. The user is anesthetized physically and does not experience much in the way of pain. As the euphoria lifts, if the user becomes paranoid and strikes out, because he feels no pain, the user is capable of inflicting a great deal more damage on others than might otherwise be the case (3,4).

CASE 15-1

Tina, age 26, had been smoking bottles of PCP for several years now. For how many years, she couldn't really remember. Actually, should truth be known, she couldn't remember much of anything. A day hadn't gone by in a long, long time that she hadn't used. Now, she had no choice. She couldn't afford it anymore. Her mother, her primary source of support, was tired of it. The authorities were threatening to take her children because her infant, born 6 months ago, had PCP in him at birth. She was so irritable, however, and every fiber was on edge when she didn't use. Of course, when she was using, she could be pretty bad too. She had put holes in the walls with her fist and broken her wrist when she was high and didn't know the bone was broken. Later, it was kind of weird to ask where the hole came from and have everyone tell her she put it there. Group therapy was really frustrating. They seemed to be on her all the time and accused her of lying when she said she didn't remember being told the rules or being confronted on specific issues. Besides, she was so depressed. She just felt like crying all the time. She didn't have any energy and everyone was against her.

Concrete descriptions are lacking of what PCP users look like or how they react in the long term. The number of PCP users has not been of the magnitude of the users of other drugs of abuse and, therefore, not warranted as much attention. One thing that has received some attention, however, is the memory problems that accompany PCP use and seriously complicate treatment. As in Tina's case, long-time heavy users of PCP appear to have profound memory deficits, having difficulty retaining information even from one day to the next. Data and experience with this population show that this effect is not permanent, although it can last for many weeks or months after cessation of use (4,5). This means that helping the patient to establish goals, develop a mechanism for acquiring and maintaining abstinence, and to devise a strategy to prevent relapse is rendered extremely difficult. Recognizing that the PCP user may not recall what has been said, it may be necessary to have the patient write everything down and review it often. The approach to the PCP user may need to be similar to the approach that would be taken with an individual with Alzheimer's disease: concrete, much repetition, in writing, and simple.

What about detoxification from PCP? In general, no detoxification from this agent is necessary. The effects will wear off over the next few hours and the patient will appear depressed and irritable or simply normal. In the case of the frightened psychotic patient requiring hospitalization, a host of papers have described the value of administering ascorbic acid to the patient, providing a quiet, nonthreatening environment, and giving alternating haloperidol and lorazepam, if necessary, to calm the patient (6–8).

Ascorbic acid, orally or intravenously, is used to acidify the urine and speed up passage of the drug from the body. PCP is excreted primarily in the urine and, as a base, is removed more quickly in an acid environment. Further, in long-term, heavy users of PCP, renal failure has been reported when hydration and acidification of the urine did not occur (9,10). Experience shows, however, that the patient who is in such great distress as a result of PCP use is unlikely to sit still for either oral or intravenous administration of vitamin C, so that this intervention, although helpful, may not be a viable option. Further, although studies from two decades ago showed some improvement in symptoms of psychosis with administration of haloperidol, data are lacking that show this medication actually decreases the period of time the patient is psychotic. In addition, the risk always exists that the patient will actually become more agitated with this approach because of the emergence of extrapyramidal side effects.

An additional issue in Tina's case is that of how her drug use may have affected her newborn. Her baby was born with this drug in its system. By her own report, she has rarely been without PCP. Thus, it can be assumed the neonate experienced heavy exposure throughout gestation. No description is given regarding delivery, birthweight, or size, thus no prediction can be made based on information about the infant itself. Further, little data are available on babies exposed the PCP. Some reviews show a substantial percentage, but less than half, of PCP babies to be small for gestational age, but further developmental data are lacking. Thus, no predictions can be made regarding how well Tina's child will do in the future (11,12).

What of the depression she describes? As is always the case, the issue of suicidal ideation and intent must be pursued so that the patient's safety can be assured. Once this is addressed, it will be nearly impossible to determine whether the depression is primary or secondary. First, it is unlikely that Tina, with her current memory deficits, could give a reliable and coherent history. Second, even if the depression is a result of the substance use, it will continue well beyond the period of discontinuation, making the distinction unimportant. Regardless of its cause, the depression will be real, uncomfortable, protracted, and have a significant impact on the patient's quality of life. Every effort should be made to find an effective treatment for her problem.

Regarding medication to treat her depression, this is an area where hard data are lacking and anecdotal and personal experience prevails. Because of the anticholinergic properties of this class of medications and the risk of further contributing to the patient's already substantial confusion, it is reasonable to avoid tricyclic antidepressants to the extent possible. PCP can induce seizures in its own right. As bupropion also lowers the seizure threshold, it would seem reasonable to avoid this medication as well.

Venlafaxine, mirtazapine, and nefazodone are all options for Tina. It should be noted, however, that it is not uncommon when people are under legal pressure to give up street drugs for them to turn to legal drugs for comfort. Because alcohol is the only legal drug available to Tina, if she does use it, medications with hepatic metabolism (e.g., venlafaxine, nefazodone) might be best avoided or used only with great caution.

Finally, simply because they have the longest track record of use and safety, it is best to try a serotonin reuptake inhibitor (SSRI) to treat this patient's condition. Although concrete studies are not available to support this approach, experience with the population has shown it to be helpful.

CASE 15-2

At 28 years of age, Katie has used so many drugs and in so many ways she really has lost count. She started at 15 years of age with speed—they used to inject that. She tried a little acid and alcohol, of course. Heroin just made her sick to her stomach. You could keep that stuff. Ecstasy was fun. You could use it a few times, walk away from it for a few days, then use it again. Cocaine and speed were the things she enjoyed most. It seemed as though she always came back to them. Katie had to admit it was difficult to finish college when you were wasted half the time, but she got it done. It was hard, but she did it. Now, she looked around and it seemed like everybody she knew had something more in their lives than she was capable of achieving. She knew she couldn't have anything and keep up the life she was leading. Besides, it wasn't fun anymore. All she did was cry, even if she was using. She wouldn't kill herself—she had put her family through enough pain. Katie had been clean except for a couple of brief slips for 4 months when she sought help for her depression. If anything, being clean made things worse. Before, she could at least look forward to something—getting high. Now nothing was fun.

As with Tina, Katie's condition will be difficult to treat, although for different reasons. Just as with Tina, it is unlikely the clinician will be able to determine with any degree of accuracy whether the depression is primary or secondary. The distinction probably is not important. Katie started using a wide variety of substances at a time when many young women begin to experience some symptoms of depression. Further, she has preferentially gravitated toward substances that, once they wear off, result in symptoms of depression, although such should be temporary.

Yet, what is temporary? Here again is an area where research is unable to give the clinician good data with which to predict a time course for recovery. In addition, Katie has used so many drugs that one might influence how the other one affects her. It is not possible to know. Further complicating the issue is that Katie has used ecstasy and methamphetamine (speed). Both of these agents cause changes in the serotonergic system during the time the drug is being used. Some evidence indicates that these agents can cause long-term neurologic changes as well (13–19). If this is the case, her depression may be caused, or seriously affected by, alterations in this part of her nervous system. Further, as research suggests, if one or both of these drugs do permanent damage to this part of the nervous system, her depression may be very difficult to treat.

Further evaluation should be done before deciding to treat Katie's depression. Is she going to be in an environment that will be conducive to her maintaining any abstinence? What is she doing to achieve this? What changes has she made in her lifestyle to make this possible? Is she developing a peer group that is not part of the drug culture? If she is not doing any of these things, it is unlikely she will be able to stay drug free. With the drugs she prefers, it will be difficult to assess whether her depression is responding to medication or constantly present because of ongoing drug use.

Unlike the case with Tina, it does not appear that anything is cognitively wrong with Katie. She was able to complete a degree program in college. She has no complaints of memory difficulties. Nevertheless, it would be helpful to ask some questions specific for cognitive functioning. The Mini-Mental State Examination might be sufficient for this purpose. No indication appears to exist for formal neurocognitive testing. With her extensive drug history, a little extra care is in order to assess for more extensive deficits.

Next is the issue of how to treat her depression. Experience with patients such as Katie shows that trial and error is the only approach. Each patient with a multidrug history of this nature is unique and the changes that may have arisen as a result of that drug history will depend on the combination of drugs that the particular patient used. It would seem obvious in Katie's case, given her extensive history of use of drugs that affect the serotonin system, to try an agent that affects this system. In her case, sertraline (200 mg) was sufficient to substantially improve her symptoms. Compare Katie's response to that of Greg, now 36 years of age, with a similar drug use history.

CASE 15-3

At 19 years of age, after a 2-week binge of methamphetamine use, Greg was brought to the emergency room accompanied by his parents and several police officers. He was combative, agitated, and convinced that the FBI and the CIA were "out to get" him. Five months and a half dozen major tranquilizers later, Greg walked out of the hospital without any medications. Nothing they gave him seemed to make any real difference—only time seemed to quiet his paranoia. Two decades later he had seen a lot of psychiatrists. He tried several antidepressants for the sad emptiness he felt, and a couple of low-dose antipsychotics for the anger he experienced in crowds and the thought that they were laughing at him when strangers smiled in his direction. Nothing had really helped however.

In Greg's case, a list was made of the symptoms that bothered him most: sadness, sleep problems, social anxiety. Then a second list was developed: suspiciousness, anger. Together, patient and physician decided on a systematic approach to the depressive features with the understanding that if the paranoia worsened, an antipsychotic would be added. Failing the newer antidepressants, Greg responded well to treatment with amoxapine. This particular medication is a tricyclic antidepressant but, as a metabolite of the antipsychotic loxapine, it has a strong dopaminergic effect as well.

Whether Greg's particularly difficult-to-treat depression is the result of permanent damage caused by long-term methamphetamine use cannot be proved. It is not uncommon, however, for clinician's to struggle to find the right medication or combination of medications to treat the psychiatric symptoms of former heavy polysubstance users such as Greg. No firm guidelines are known to steer the clinician in the treatment of the depressed polydrug user. A systematic trial of agents for reasonable periods of time is a necessary approach.

CASE 15-4

When his brother brought Ted M., 23 years of age, to the doctor, it was hard to tell who was more frightened and upset—his brother or him. He kept seeing—well—things. Sometimes, it was silly things like teddy bears and bubbles; sometimes, terrifying things like skulls and arms with huge swords that suddenly appeared threatening to slash his throat. He hadn't used any drugs in more than 5 days, but things weren't getting any better. There was that deep voice too, only now it was threatening him. The bubbles and skulls were new but the voice—he couldn't remember how long it had been with him—at least a year, maybe more. As he told the doctor these things, the tears poured. He had spent a long weekend with friends, he related. They had used a variety of drugs— nitrous oxide, alcohol, ice—he couldn't really remember what all there had been. But that ended 5 days ago, and these visions and voices had not. Drug binges like that weren't new for him. He'd started using substances in middle school, huffing butane with his friends. He came slowly into the room with his head down, the psychomotor retardation of depression obvious. As he sat, every now and then an arm or leg would twitch or his head would suddenly move. He did not seem to be aware of these movements.

Again, this patient is going to be a diagnostic dilemma and difficult to treat. Exactly what is wrong with the young man? It would be simple to say that his is a substance-induced psychosis, but what of the auditory hallucinations that he has had for more than a year? Both short- and long-term issues need to be addressed.

First, is the issue of the patient's immediate comfort and safety. Should he be hospitalized? If he has a supportive environment, does not wish to be in the foreign environment of the hospital, and can contract for safety, it may be possible for him to have out-patient treatment. After all, he has been suffering from this for 5 days outside the confines of the hospital.

What to give him is a bit confusing. It is not at all clear what is giving him this reaction. The time course of the reaction is unusual. In most cases, by 5 days an acute psychotic reaction to most drugs should be resolving. It would appear that Ted M. is going to be a patient who, if the problem is a drug-induced psychosis, is in for a much more protracted course than if he had a more typical psychotic reaction.

A substantial body of older research literature is available regarding the treatment of substance-induced psychosis; however, controlled studies are lacking (20,21). Whereas anecdotal reports favor one or another typical antipsychotic medication for ameliorating the positive symptoms the patient experiences, meta-analysis and personal experience provide little evidence that such is of much benefit. Nevertheless, when a patient is in this much distress, compelling reasons exist to do something, as opposed to nothing.

New reports are emerging regarding the utility of the newer antipsychotics for treating such patients. Again, controlled studies are lacking, but it is possible the atypical antipsychotics may be more beneficial. In addition, the lower risk of akathisia, which could increase the patient's already substantial anxiety, makes using an atypical antipsychotic preferable.

This particular patient received risperidone, although quetiapine, olanzapine, or ziprasidone might also have been tried. Because of the need to have patients on the clozapine registry and to have blood work performed and reviewed before receiving clozapine, this is not an agent to consider in a "hurry up" situation.

What about the apparent depression and psychomotor retardation Ted is displaying? It is actually too soon to be able to judge with any certainty what is going on in this regard and, with his safety assured, no reason is seen to rush to treat this symptom. His greatest source of distress is the psychosis, the frightening visual hallucinations, and this should be the target symptom. It is common for inhalant users to demonstrate depressive symptoms, although this often appears to be time limited. Ted indicates he began "huffing" (i.e., using inhalants) as a young teen. In addition, he had used nitrous oxide, also an inhalant, as recently as 5 days before his visit to his doctor. This could be sufficient to explain his depressed appearance. He also used "ice" (methamphetamine) during his drug binge. Just as with cocaine, a depression follows a binge on this drug. Perhaps this could partially account for his presentation. Time will tell.

Ted's history of beginning to use inhalant drugs in his early teens is not unusual. This is the typical time for onset of such drug use. Further, such drug use is much more common than many people think. According to the National Institute on Drug

Abuse, nearly a fifth of all eighth graders have used inhalants. The fact that some of these substances can cause long-term neuronal damage makes this a particularly frightening statistic.

This long-term or perhaps permanent neuronal damage may account for Ted's twitches. Long-term users of inhalants can develop neurologic damage as a result of demyelination resulting in abnormal gait or movements. It is possible that this is what the observer was seeing, although it may simply be too soon to tell with this acutely ill young man.

CASE 15-5

One year after Ted M.'s initial presentation, he still experienced auditory hallucinations. It had been learned that Ted had a family history of alcohol dependence in the paternal grandfather and a paternal uncle. No other psychiatric history was found on either side of the family, however. Specifically, no family history of psychosis existed of which anyone was aware. During that year, Ted had been poorly compliant with his medication. Although the risperidone was successful in helping him to rest and ridded him of the visual hallucinations, the voices never really left him. Several other antipsychotics provided similar symptom relief. Despite the benefits, Ted was resistive to the idea of staying on medications, although he was unable to verbalize why other than to state he did not feel he needed them. Each time he discontinued antipsychotic treatment, however, he became withdrawn, disheveled, and marginally functional. Family members related that he rarely bathed or came out of his room, and could be heard talking to himself at night behind closed doors when not medicated.

Now what is the diagnosis for Ted's condition and what is to be done about it? The current description sounds like schizophrenia. In addition, he responds well to antipsychotic medication, although incompletely so. Does this mean he has schizophrenia and will likely need medication long term? Or does the incompleteness of his response mean he has a substance-induced psychosis and can be expected eventually to be relieved of all symptoms and off all medications?

The answer is, no answer exists. It is not possible to predict with any degree of certainty what will happen with Ted. What is clear is that he will require much support and encouragement to remain on medication because he does not do well without it at this point. Further, the longer he remains substance free, the easier it will be to gauge exactly what is happening to him mentally.

REFERENCES

1. McCardle L, Fishbein DH. The self-reported effects of PCP on human aggression. *Addict Behav* 1989;14(4):465–472.
2. Brecher M, Wang B, Wong H, et al. Phencyclidine and violence: clinical and legal issues. *J Clin Psychopharmacol* 1988;8(6):397–401.
3. Julien RM. *A primer of drug action.* New York: WH Freeman, 1997.

4. Infofax N. *PCP (phencyclidine)*. Bethesda, MD: National Institute on Drug Abuse, 2001:2.

5. Cosgrove J, Newell TG. Recovery of neuropsychological functions during reduction in use of phencyclidine. *J Clin Psychol* 1991;47(1):159–169.

6. Giannini AJ, Eighan MS, Loiselle RH, et al. Comparison of haloperidol and chlorpromazine in the treatment of phencyclidine psychosis. *J Clin Pharmacol* 1984;24:202–204.

7. Lvisada PV, Brown BI. Clinical management of the phencyclidine psychosis. *Clin Toxicol* 1976;9(4):539–545.

8. Perez-Reyes M, DiGuiseppi S, Brine DR, et al. Urine pH and phencyclidine excretion. *Clin Pharmacol Ther* 1982;32:635–641.

9. Simpson GM, Khajawall AM, Alatorre E, et al. Urinary phencyclidine excretion in chronic abusers. *J Toxicol Clin Toxicol* 1982–1983;19(10):1051–1059.

10. Patel R, Connor G. Review of thirty cases of rhabdomyolysis associated acute renal failure among phencyclidine users. *J Toxicol Clin Toxicol* 1985–1986;23(7–8):547–556.

11. Golden NL, Kuhnert BR, Sokol RJ, et al. Phencyclidine use during pregnancy. *Am J Obstet Gynecol* 1984;148:254–259.

12. Rahbar F, Famufod A, White D, et al. Impact of intrauterine exposure to phencyclidine (PCP) and cocaine on neonates. *J Natl Med Assoc* 1993;85:349–352.

13. Rodgers J. Cognitive performance amongst recreational users of "ecstasy." *Psychopharmacology* 2000;151(1):19–24.

14. Buffenstein A, Heaster J, Ko P. Chronic psychotic illness from methamphetamine. *Am J Psychiatry* 1999;156(4):662.

15. Croft RJ, Klugman A, Baldeweg T, et al. Electrophysiological evidence of serotonergic impairment in long term MDMA users. *Am J Psychiatry* 2001;158(10):1687–1692.

16. Ernst T, Chang L, Leonido-Yee M, et al. Evidence for long-term neurotoxicity associated with methamphetamine abuse. *Neurology* 2000;54(6):1344–1349.

17. Fox HC, Parrott AC, Turner JJ. Ecstasy use: cognitive deficits related to dosage rather than self-reported problematic use of the drug. *J Psychopharmacol* 2001;15(4):273–281.

18. MacInnes N, Handley SL, Harding GF. Former chronic MDMA users report mild depressive symptoms. *J Psychopharmacol* 2001; 15(3):181–186.

19. McCann UD, Ricaurte GA, Molliver ME. "Ecstasy" and serotonin neurotoxicity. *Arch Gen Psychiatry* 2001;58(10):907–908.

20. Misra LK, Kofoed L, Oesterheld JR, et al. Olanzapine treatment of methamphetamine psychosis. *J Clin Psychopharmacol* 2000; 20(3):393–394.

21. Srisurapanont M, Kittiratanapaiboon P, Jarusuraisin N. Treatment for amphetamine psychosis [review]. *Cochrane Database Syst Rev* 2001.

Treating the Dually Diagnosed

A PROGRAM FOR THE DUALLY DIAGNOSED

1. Following assumptions are made
   a. Both psychiatric and substance use disorder have remissions and exacerbations
      i. Psychiatric condition must be stable enough for the patient and others to be safe
      ii. Patient must be out of danger of withdrawal
   b. Patient must have some degree of engagement in program
2. Clinician will try to help the patient find a reason to stay in treatment
3. Program elements
   a. What does the patient expect as a result of using
      i. Help patients focus on what they desire to get from using versus what actually happens
      ii. Identify alternative means of receiving these desired benefits
      iii. Some patients identify genuine positives to using (e.g., cocaine and negative symptoms of schizophrenia)
         (a) Deal with these honestly
         (b) Search for alternatives
   b. Helping the patient identify symptoms of illness
      i. Patients may have no idea of what constitutes normalcy
      ii. Helping the patient recognize signs and symptoms of illness also helps the patient seek intervention before significant worsening
      iii. Clinician must try to understand how patients feel about a particular symptom: not all patients perceive all symptoms as negative
   c. Identifying things to do when symptoms worsen
      i. Empowers or gets the patient prepared ahead of time
      ii. Make a list of possibilities ahead of time
      iii. Have the patient keep the list of possibilities on his or her person and practice them ahead of time
   d. Medication education
      i. Patients often have no idea of the purpose of their medications
      ii. Factual information about medications permits patients to make informed choices regarding how and if they will take medications as well as whether they will mix them with substances of abuse
      iii. Factual information is given about interaction between medications and substances of abuse

Attachments. Handouts for patients to use in program

In the preceding chapters were discussed evaluation of the dually diagnosed patient, detoxification from various substances of abuse, how comorbid conditions affect each other, and issues to consider when choosing a medication for treating comorbid conditions. This chapter presents materials that can be used by patients themselves. Throughout the chapters emphasis is that patients often need help finding a reason to stay in treatment, that the more they understand about themselves and their illnesses, the better they can equip themselves to avoid succumbing to either the substance use disorder or to the mental illness (Figs. 16-1 and 16-2). This

Please think of reasons you might not attend this program. If some of these reasons are

identified in the list below, please check off all reasons that apply to you. Add any other reasons

you can think of for not attending.

Reasons not to attend:
1. It's boring
2. I don't want to listen to other people's problems
3. I'll be hassled about drinking and drugging
4. Other people will be telling me what to do
5. None of this stuff ever works for me
6. I don't have a mental illness so I shouldn't be here
7. I'm not going to quit drugging/drinking so why should I be here?
8. I don't like the people here
9. I think the things that are done or discussed are silly
10. I wouldn't come if I wasn't forced to, so I probably won't get anything out of it
11. I don't have a drinking/drugging problem so why should I be here?
12. Nobody here has the same types of problems I have
13. I don't believe in God or a higher power and that's all they talk about
14. Other (please list)
15.
16.
17.

Figure 16-1.

chapter contains handouts used by dually diagnosed clients, as
well as explanations and examples of how each can be used to help
dually diagnosed patients help themselves. Some materials, for example, the "Substance Checklist" (Figs. 16-3 through 16-7) have
proved valuable for working with substance-abusing patients who
are not mentally ill as well. Others, such as the "Symptom Checklist" (Fig. 16-8), are specific to dually diagnosed individuals. They
are designed to help them recognize symptoms of their illnesses
and to identify what to do about them when they worsen. Some patients (e.g., those with schizophrenia) may require much repetition
and reminders of how their mental illness and substance use can
affect each other. Less concrete thinkers, on the other hand, may
grasp the concepts quickly and move on.

Materials presented here are used with the assumption that
most of the treatment occurs in the context of group work. The

Please think of reasons you might attend this program. If some of these reasons are identified in the list below, please check off all reasons that apply to you. Add any other reasons you can think of for attending.

	Reasons to attend:
	1. Charges will be dropped
	2. People may understand me here
	3. It's someplace to go and something to do
	4. Maybe this will help, since I want to stop using but can't
	5. Maybe I'll be able to control my mental illness better
	6. I like being here
	7. My family/friends will be pleased
	8. The voices are not as loud when I'm around other people
	9. I'm not sure, but I might get something out of it
	10. I think there's something wrong with me and maybe I'll find out what if I come
	11. I hope I can learn to control my drinking or drugging
	12. Maybe I can help someone else here who has problems like I have or had
	13. Other (please list):
	14.
	15.
	16.

Figure 16-2.

high cost of individual therapy and the relative lack of treatment providers available to work with the dually diagnosed make it necessary to approach several dually diagnosed patients at once. These same materials have been successfully adapted to individual and couples work, however.

Other assumptions are also made. First, it is assumed that the patient's psychiatric condition is relatively stable and that patient and staff can feel safe in the treatment environment. Exacerbations and remissions will occur in the condition that will have a strong impact on how the patient responds to the various interventions. Every effort is made to ensure the patient is as stable at any one time as is possible, however.

It is also assumed that the patient will have periods of relapses and remission in substance use. Relapse is used as a learning tool and not necessarily a cause for discharge. As long as it is felt that

(text continues on page 194)

MARIJUANA CHECKLIST

When I use marijuana, I feel: (Check all that apply)		While the marijuana is working I: (Please check all that apply)		After I use marijuana: (Check all that apply to you)		After reviewing your list, in general does using marijuana give you what you're looking for?		
						Yes	No	Not sure
Mellow	Drowsy	Feel different (good)	Feel sleepy	I feel tired	More paranoid	If it does, can you think of other ways of getting what you're looking for? (Make a list)		
Like everybody else	Different	Feel different (bad)	Fit in better	I feel happy	Need less medicine			
Normal	More energetic	Get less paranoid	Eat more	I get less paranoid	End up in the hospital less often			
Happy	Calm	Feel more mellow	Feel Happy	Nothing changes	Don't have any energy			
Less paranoid	Like I fit in	Feel more alert	Get more paranoid	I feel suicidal	Sleep better			
Nothing in particular, I just like it	Silly	Can't think straight	Hear voices less	I feel more energetic	Can't sleep well			
More sensitive to others	Numb	My heart pounds	Don't feel any different	I feel depressed	I hear voices more	If it doesn't, what can you do that will get you what you want? (List)		
More aware of my surroundings	Hear voices more	Hear voices more	Don't care about things	Need more medicine	Don't have any energy			
Like my thoughts are slower	I sleep better	Feel more tense	Feel smarter	I end up in the hospital more often	I sleep better			
Like I can think better	Less depressed	Relate better to others	Feel depressed	I get angry more easily	I can't sleep well			
Other (list)		Can think better	Eat less	Act silly				
		Feel numb		Other				
		Other (list)						

Figure 16-3.

ALCOHOL CHECKLIST

When I use alcohol, I want to feel: (Check all that apply)		When I use alcohol (that is while it's working): (Check all that apply to you)		After I use alcohol, that is after it has worn off, I feel: (Check all that apply to you)		After reviewing your list, in general, does using alcohol give you what you're looking for?		
						Yes	No	Not sure
More energetic	Happy	Different (good)	More energetic	Sad	Fine	If yes, it does, can you think of other ways of getting what you're looking for that won't get you into trouble with the law, your family, etc.? (Make a list)		
Like I fit in	Sleepy	Sleepy	Like people are watching me	Like I need to have less medicine	More depressed			
Like nothing matters	Different	Suicidal	Like I do dumb things	Less paranoid	A bad headache			
Nothing in particular, I just like it	More Sociable	Tired	Like dancing	More paranoid	Suicidal			
Numb	Silly	Like laughing	Like nothing matters	No different	Let down			
Other (list)		More depressed	Less paranoid	Sleepy	Less depressed			
		Different (bad)	Less depressed	Tired	Happy	If it doesn't, what can you do that will get you what you want? (Make a list)		
		Like the voices are softer	Like I am going to get sick	Ashamed	Like I have to have more medicine			
		Like I can't think as well	Can talk to people more easily	Other (make a list)				
		Like the voices are louder	Like the room is spinning					
		Like being around people	Don't feel any different					
		Like avoiding people	Can think better					
		More paranoid	Like crying					
		Other (make a list)						

Figure 16-4.

"OTHER" CHECKLIST

When I use ____, I want to feel: (Check all that apply)	When I use ____ (that is while it's working) I feel: (Check all that apply to you)		After I use ____ (Check all that apply to you)	____ that is after it has worn off, I feel:	After reviewing your list, in general, does using ____ give you what you're looking for?		
	Different (good)	More energetic		Fine	Yes	No	Not sure
Happy					**If yes, it does, can you think of other ways of getting what you're looking for that won't get you into trouble with the law, your family, etc.? (Make a list)**		
Sleepy	Sleepy	Like people are watching me	Ashamed	More depressed			
Different	Suicidal	Like I do dumb things	More paranoid	A bad headache			
More Sociable	Tired	Like dancing	No different	Suicidal			
Silly	Like laughing	Like nothing matters	Sick to my stomach	Let down			
Numb	More depressed	Less paranoid	Sad	Less depressed			
Nothing in particular, I just like it	Different (bad)	Less depressed	Like I need to have less medicine	Happy			
More energetic	Voices are softer	Other (make a list)	Less paranoid	Like I have to have more medicine			
Like I fit in	Can't think as well	Like crying	Tired	Sleepy	**If it doesn't, what can you do that will get you what you want? (Make a list)**		
Like nothing matters	Like the voices are louder	Sometimes, like I am going to get sick	Other				
Other:	Like being around people	Like I can talk to people more easily					
	Like avoiding people	Sometimes like the room is spinning					
	More paranoid	Don't feel any different					

Figure 16-5.

HEROIN CHECKLIST

When I use heroin, I want to feel: (Check all that apply)	When I use heroin, that is while it's working, I feel: (Check all that apply to you)	After I use heroin, that is after it has worn off, I feel: (Check all that apply to you)	After reviewing your list, in general, does using heroin give you what you're looking for?		
			Yes	No	Not sure
Mellow	Mellow	Fine	If yes, it does, can you think of other ways of getting what you're looking for that won't get you into trouble with the law, your family, etc.? (Make a list)		
Drowsy	Calmer	More depressed			
Different	Sexy	A bad headache			
High	Sleepy	Suicidal			
Numb	More paranoid	Let down			
Like everybody else	More tense	Less depressed			
Sexy	Numb	Happy			
Calmer	Like no one can hurt me	Like I have to have more medicine			
Other	Like people want to hurt me	Sleepy			
	Different	Tired			
	Less paranoid	Ashamed	If it doesn't, what can you do that will get you what you want? (Make a list)		
	Like I have to watch people	More paranoid			
	More alert	No different			
	Other (make a list)	Sick to my stomach			
		Sad			
		Like I need to have less medicine			
		Less paranoid			
		Other			

Figure 16-6.

COCAINE CHECKLIST

When I use cocaine, I want to feel: (Check all that apply)	When I use cocaine (that is, while it's working) I feel: (Please check all that apply)		After I use cocaine: (Check all that apply to you)		After reviewing your list, in general, does using cocaine give you what you're looking for?		
					Yes	No	Not sure
Happy	Better	Paranoid	I feel energetic	I feel happy			
Like everybody else	Worse	Different (good)	I am depressed	I feel suicidal			
Like the voices are quieter	Weird	Different (bad)	I end up in the hospital	I feel tired			
Energetic	Calmer	Like I can think better	I feel rested	I can't sleep			
Sexy	More jittery	The voices get softer	I'm hospitalized less often	I sleep too much			
Manic	The same	Sexy	Nothing changes	I have fewer legal problems			
Different than usual	Angry	Like I can't breathe	I have ended up in jail	I don't need as much medicine			
Nothing particular, I just like it	Like I'm going too fast	I start sweating	I feel ashamed	My family/ friends get angry with me			
Like my thoughts are slower	Like everybody else	Like people are watching me	I am more paranoid	I feel like people are looking at me			
Better than usual	Like I can't think straight	Sometimes I get a headache	I need more medicine	Family/ friends are pleased with me			
High	The voices get louder	I have gotten into fights	Other:				
Calm	Like someone's trying to hurt me	Sick to my stomach					
Other:	Pain in my chest	Suspicious of people					
	My heart pounding						

Are there other ways of getting what you're looking for that won't get you into trouble with the law, your family, etc.? Such as: (check all that apply)

Figure 16-7.

SYMPTOM CHECKLIST										
SYMPTOM	HOW I FEEL ABOUT IT								THINGS THAT MAKE IT WORSE	THINGS THAT MAKE IT BETTER
	Good	Bad	Neutral	Angry	Sad	Happy	Scared	Other		
I hear things other people don't appear to hear										
I see things other people don't appear to see										
Something/someone is taking thoughts out of my head										
The radio and/ or TV talk directly to me										
I intentionally hurt myself by burning myself or cutting on myself										
I have, or have thought I had, special powers										
I talk so fast other people can't understand me										
My thoughts go so fast I can't follow them										
My thoughts confuse me										
I feel like people want to hurt me										
I have tried to kill myself										
I hear people talking when there isn't anyone around										
I feel like people are watching me										
Someone/something is controlling my thoughts or actions										
The newspaper writes articles directly to me										

Figure 16-8a.

SYMPTOM CHECKLIST

SYMPTOM	HOW I FEEL ABOUT IT								THINGS THAT MAKE IT WORSE	THINGS THAT MAKE IT BETTER
	Good	Bad	Neutral	Angry	Sad	Happy	Scared	Other		
I have tried to hurt other people when I thought they were mocking me or that they might hurt me										
I believe or have believed that I am someone others say I'm not										
People tell me I talk too fast										
I have done things or said things when I was going too fast that I didn't mean to do										
I feel like people are following me										
Sometimes I think I'm crazy										
I have trouble getting to sleep										
Something/someone is putting thoughts into my head										
I have gone on spending sprees buying things I didn't need when I was going too fast										
I want to hurt people										
I cry a lot										
I get angry easily										
I have trouble breathing when I am in a crowd										
Sometimes I feel like I'm going to die										

Figure 16-8b.

Sometimes my heart starts pounding for no reason																
I have trouble staying asleep																
*I am seriously thinking about hurting myself or killing myself right now																
I want to kill people																
I cry for no reason																
Memories I want to forget come suddenly into my mind																
I have trouble breathing when I am in a strange situation																
Sometimes I feel like I'm not here at all																
I feel like the walls are closing in on me																

*An answer that this is the case is clearly cause for the therapist to stop the proceedings and assess the client for potential lethality

Figure 16-8c.

the patient is making progress and improving self, psychiatric condition, and substance use problem, the patient is welcome to stay in the treatment program. Discharge occurs when violence or threats of violence occur or if it is felt that the program and its components are not of benefit to the patient.

It is also assumed that the patient is detoxified from the substance of abuse and using no more frequently than on an occasional basis. That is, the threat of significant withdrawal symptoms is absent.

In the treatment program, six basic issues comprise the subject of focus. Each may have to be revisited periodically, depending on the severity of the patient's psychiatric condition and the frequency with which relapse occurs. These issues are:

1. Helping the patient find a reason or goals for treatment
2. Expectations for using and realities of using substances
3. Alternatives to using
4. Identifying symptoms of illness
5. Identifying what to do when symptoms become worse
6. Understanding interactions between substances of abuse, mental illness, and medications

HELPING THE PATIENT FIND A REASON TO STAY IN TREATMENT

As noted in Chapter 3, patients come to treatment for a variety of reasons and can be less than happy to be there. They may present with a hostile attitude toward the process. Figures 1 and 2 depict an exercise designed to help the individual find a reason to stay in treatment.

The patient is encouraged to list "cons" and "pros" of participation as they apply to the patient personally, not in a global or general sense. This gets patients away from the habit of telling the treatment provider what they think the clinician wants to hear and on to solving personal problems and developing personal solutions. It is emphasized that this list be written for two reasons. First, is an effort to avoid a confrontation and digression from the exercise in the case of the patient unhappy about being in treatment. The mere fact of writing things down can often render them less important. Second, this exercise is done in a group format. Each patient is given an opportunity to offer only one item per time around the group. By moving on and giving each person a chance to speak, the attention of the angry patient is drawn onto the others and away from personal anger.

The review starts with the downside or "con" list to participation. This lets the angry or mandated patient get some hostility off his or her chest. The exercise ends with the "pro" list to become and remain focused on a more positive side. Most patients, given the opportunity to express their unhappiness at the situation, are willing to accept the possibility that something positive can come of it, although they may need help from the therapist to find what that might be.

At the end of this exercise, most patients, grudgingly perhaps, will have some reason to continue. Occasionally, patients will remain greatly opposed to continuing in treatment, even after hearing their peers gain acceptance of the idea. If this happens, it may be necessary to explore further with the patient what exactly has brought that person to therapy. If under pressure from family or the law to remain in treatment, the therapist can focus on the "pro" list, indicating the patient will have less pressure. If the patient continues to be negative or even begins to work up into an angry outburst, it is wise simply to invite the patient to "try things" for awhile and see how he or she feels about remaining after a few session (see Figures 16-1 and 16-2).

EXPECTATIONS OF SUBSTANCE USE

Next, is an exercise that helps the patient begin to focus on expectations of substance use and identify alternate ways of achieving the desired result (Figs. 16-3 through 16-7).

In this exercise, each patient is asked to fill in everything on the "Checklist" that applies to current drug use. The first set of columns asks what the patient wants the drug to do for him or her; the next set of columns asks what happens while the patient is actually using the drug. Column three asks what happens after using the particular drug. The last column deals with whether the drug did what the patient wanted it to do and alternatives for achieving the desired result.

Most patients, if they are honest with themselves, will be experiencing far more negative than positive consequences of substance use. "Coming down" and recovering from intoxication, withdrawal, and increased risk of hospitalization are all part of the down side of using. This exercise permits patients the opportunity to gently confront their use, what it is actually doing to them, and explore alternative behaviors. It is assumed that the patient has come to treatment for a reason, and the most likely being that substance use and mental disorder are causing significant difficulty in one or more aspects of his or her life.

CASE 16-1

Tim, 32, used nicotine, cocaine, alcohol, and marijuana, in that order. He smoked a joint now and then, but only to be sociable. It was always around. He drank alcohol, but only when he was using crack. Cocaine he used because it helped him think straight and talk to other people. It was one of the few times others seemed to understand what he was saying.

Tim is a patient who has identified a true benefit of his drug of choice. Having schizophrenia, he recognizes that when he uses cocaine he is more sociable and has less difficulty communicating with others. He almost feels "normal" or, at least, he is able to fit into a group better when he is using cocaine.

On his expectations list he noted the benefits of his cocaine use. He was able to recognize, however, the consequences of using as well. Assessing the issues honestly, in the third column, he indicated he recognized an increase in paranoia and an increased likelihood of hospitalization. Then, in column four, it was clear the benefit he received was very temporary. This opened the way for a conversation on other ways to achieve the benefits of using. Such strategies as trying a different medication were added to column four.

IDENTIFYING SYMPTOMS OF ILLNESS

It is not uncommon for patients, especially the young ones, to deny they have a mental illness and to deny the need for medication. They can go through repeated episodes of hospitalizations, improvements, throwing away their medications, decompensation, and hospitalization again before they finally come to accept a need for medication compliance. The same is true for substance users and, for that matter, just about every other condition. People need to prove to themselves that they truly have to do something before they do it. Take the example of the diabetic who finally decides to swear off cookies, because he simply does not feel good after he eats them and his blood sugar level is above 350. Or, consider the hypertensive who decides that the explosive headache he gets when his blood pressure is out of control is not worth the salted peanuts he ate that then pushed his pressure up so high.

It is also true that some patients simply have no idea what "normal" is. Children who need glasses for nearsightedness typically begin to do so when they are about 8 or 9 years of age. Parents are often horrified to hear their offspring exclaim about seeing individual leaves on trees, separate blades of grass, or insects on the sidewalk when they get their first set of glasses, saying they had never seen these things before. Parents often guiltily comment that they did not know the child could not see, not realizing the child did not know either. Never having seen these things before, the child could not miss them or know to tell anyone. Likewise, the individual who has quietly been carrying on a conversation with someone only he can see is justified in asking "how do I know what you can see and hear?" when asked if he hears things that others do not.

Figure 16-8 depicting the symptoms of various illnesses serves more than one purpose. The figure gently focuses the attention of the individual who is denying his or her illness and defines some of the experiences as "symptoms." It also helps the treatment provider to become familiar with what the patient is personally experiencing. Further, it reassures group members that others have and do experience many of the same problems they themselves have encountered. As new patients enter the group, old members can review and share their lists and encourage newcomers to develop and share their own. Old members often commiserate with new members and share how they endured or overcame similar symptoms. They can also be helpful to newcomers by letting them know help is available for their problem and that things can get better. Those who are very guarded, suspicious, or uncomfortable can be encouraged to remain and observe what others say and do.

CASE 16-2

Lisa, 27 years old, was always pleasant and smiling while in the group. She greeted each new person with "Jesus loves you" and would nod wisely after she said it. She would then turn to the left and mutter something behind her hand before repeating "Jesus loves you." Lisa happily related to the new doctor that, yes, a voice spoke to her constantly. It was the voice of Jesus telling her He loved her and He loved everyone. Sometimes He spoke just for her, very intimate things, but she wouldn't talk about that, she blushed. She had stopped all the cocaine and reefer, she told Him, and was doing just fine. Jesus had told her those things would

*keep her out of heaven, so she no longer used them. The doctor in-
dicated to Lisa that it seemed an increase in her medication was
indicated if she was hearing voices all the time. He handed her a
prescription and told her to come back in a week to tell him if the
problem had improved. She did not return to the program.*

As patients share what symptoms they experience or have experienced, the group leader should ask patients how they feel about
their various symptoms. Not all symptoms of major mental illness
are experienced as negative, and patients may not wish to give
them up. For example, some individuals indicate they enjoy their
auditory hallucinations and would be lonely without the voices that
talk to them. Assuming that the voices are undesirable may cause
a patient to want to hide symptoms to avoid medication changes
that might take away this source of pleasure. At any rate, it may
harm the relationship the leader is trying to develop with the patient. This is clearly what happened in Lisa's case. Had the physician listened to the message, he would have realized his patient
would have no motivation for changing her situation. She was
happy with the comforting and friendly hallucinations that made
her feel special. Further, the voice had acted in the role of moral
control and helped her to stop using drugs. Without it, did Lisa
have other skills to help her remain drug free? The physician
knows far too little about the patient and her functioning from this
interaction alone to make judgments about her needs at this juncture. Much more information should be gathered before making
significant changes in the patient's treatment (Fig. 16-8).

In addition to information about symptoms, patients should be
educated about the conditions themselves. Many people feel guilty
about taking medication "just for depression" or "just for anxiety,"
as though these conditions were not disabling or were somehow
signs of weakness. Figure 9 was developed to present concrete
information about mental illnesses. Stress is placed on the fact
that psychiatric illnesses are the result of complex neurobiological
changes and that a psychiatric illness (e.g., depression) is a "sick-
ness, not a sin." Because psychiatric disorders are physical illnesses
just as diabetes or hypertension is, they are often treated with
medication, as are diabetes and hypertension (Fig. 16-9).

THINGS TO DO WHEN SYMPTOMS GET BAD

Initially, patients may have no idea what they can do to help
themselves when their symptoms worsen. If patients are unable
to think of ways to help themselves and things that make their
symptoms better and worse, they can learn by listening to others.
Again, the intention is to empower patients to the degree possible
and to let them take as much control as is reasonable given their
mental status.

CASE 16-3

*Matthew L., 25 years of age, had been hearing voices for several
years. In the preceding months, however, they had become increasingly insistent and hostile, telling him to hit people he had never*
(text continues on page 200)

DIAGNOSIS	SYMPTOMS	MEDICATIONS
Bipolar disorders (Manic depression)	Severe mood swings – way too high or way too low	"Mood stabilizers" including valproic acid, lithium, and carbamazepine
Mania	Move too fast	May use an antipsychotic
	Talk too fast	May use an antidepressant
	Impulsive behavior	
	Heightened (high risk) sexual behavior	
	Can have delusions, especially that one has special powers	
	Decreased need for sleep	
Depression	See below	
Anxiety attacks	Increased heart rate	Benzodiazepines (should be avoided with individuals with a history of addiction)
	Shortness of breath	Buspar
	Feeling of tightness in the chest	Some tricyclic antidepressants
	Avoidance of socials situations	General: serotonin reuptake inhibitor antidepressants
	Avoidance of leaving home	
	Avoidance of any activity or situation that might cause a recurrence of these "attacks"	
	Belief that one is going to die	
	Belief that the walls are closing in	

Depression	Depressed mood	Antidepressants
	Easy/frequent tearfulness	Mood stabilizers
	Anger out of proportion to events	Shock treatments if not responding to other activities
	Wishing one would die	Combinations of medications including hormones
	Thoughts of or plans for suicide	
	Decreased or increased appetite	
	Decreased or increased sleep	
	Decreased or increased non-directed activity	
	Decreased sex drive	
Schizophrenia	Paranoia	Antipsychotics
	Auditory or visual hallucinations	May add "mood stabilizer"
	Feelings that the TV or radio is giving one special messages	Combinations of medications
	Feeling that someone or something is putting thoughts into one's head	
	Feeling that someone or something is taking thoughts out of one's head	
	Delusions	
	Thought blocking – where just don't seem to be able to think at all	
	Inability to feel any emotions	

Figure 16-9.

seen before and other things of that nature. He told the group the voice was becoming harder to ignore, but he didn't want to act on its instructions. Another patient, a veteran of the group, offered: "when those voices start telling me to do things, I just turn around and tell them "no" and then I come here." Matthew hadn't realized he could tell a voice "no" and indicated he would try this.

A recurrent theme that must be heard by patients, regardless of diagnosis, is the necessity of avoiding isolating themselves. As they begin to feel worse, patients tend to withdraw. They need to understand that this is precisely the time they need others the most. The patient who offered that he came here (to the program) had clearly heard this message.

Finally, for the patients who seem to be stuck, a checklist is included to help get them going on ways to help themselves when things are difficult symptomatically (Fig. 16-10).

WHAT MEDICATIONS ARE SUPPOSED TO DO FOR PATIENTS

Patients often have misconceptions of what medications are supposed to do for them. As noted elsewhere, patient noncompliance with medication is a major factor in relapse to psychiatric symptoms. Effort is made to educate the patient to what medications do and do not do. In addition, the patient's resistance to taking medication is explored. Figure 16-11 depicts an exercise developed to look at reasons against and for taking medications. Patients are asked to fill it out for themselves, then to read and discuss their answers with the group. Often peer feedback can be very valuable (Fig. 16-11).

CASE 16-4

John, 25, had a list "against" taking medications that was quite a bit longer than his list "for." It included not needing it, feeling happier without it, and not wanting to be told what to do. He had been attending clinic for a couple of months, court-mandated to treatment as an alternative to jail. Helen, another patient, started laughing. "When you first came in here nobody could understand a thing you said because you didn't make sense. You talked all nonsense. You're on medication now and everybody knows what you're saying. I won't tell you what to do, but you'll go back to being the fool if you stop that stuff now." John became angry and started to argue. Helen's words weren't exactly soothing. She started imitating his behavior from early on in his time in group and got him laughing, however. Fortunately, John was able to see the humor in the mimicry and entered into the spirit of the exercise.

Once the patients have had a chance to express their likes and dislikes, the clinician can offer concrete information on the purpose of the medications and what they can and cannot do. In addition, suggestions can be made for how to counter the negatives of the medication when they arise (Figs. 16-12 and 16-13).

(text continues on page 205)

Things to do when the symptoms get bad (check all you think might be helpful to you)		
Call someone (Phone no.:)	Listen to the radio	Practice relaxation exercises
Go to a 12-step meeting (Address:)	Read a book	Take a shower
Call the clinic (Phone no.:)	Call a family member (phone no:)	Tell the voice no
Come to the program (Address:)	Go for a walk	Make a list of things you like
Write down a list of things that make you smile	Write down a list of things that seem calm	Other
Other	Other	

Figure 16-10.

People have different reasons for choosing to take or not take medication. What have been your reasons for taking or not taking medications prescribed for you? Please check all that apply.

MEDICATIONS: Reasons to take or not take medications

Reasons to not take			Reasons to take					
Reason	PAST	NOW	Reason	PAST	NOW	Reason	PAST	NOW
I get too sleepy			Feel more relaxed			Voices are quieter or stop		
Makes me confused			I feel happier			In jail less often		
Less comfortable with people			Makes thoughts clearer			Concentration improved		
Can't concentrate			I'm friendlier			In hospital less often		
Get tight muscles			Talk to people more easily			Get along better with people		
Thirsty all the time			Can sleep better			Less paranoid		
Feel "wired"								
Can't relax								
Gain weight			I feel less anxious			Less depressed		
Get movements I can't control			Don't get bad thoughts			Don't have to hurt myself		
Can't sit still			Feel calmer			I'm less frightened		
Makes me nervous inside or jittery								
I drool								
Have to walk all the time								
Makes me too tired								
Feel sad with medication								
Trouble having sex								
Can't mix with alcohol/other drugs								
Have to go to clinic all the time								
Don't need medication								
Other:			Other:			Other:		

Figure 16-11.

MEDICATIONS: WHAT THEY DO

Medication family	Example	Illnesses treated	Target symptoms	Interaction with alcohol/other drugs	Possible problems	Possible remedies
Major tranquilizers	Clozapine (clozaril)	Schizophrenia	Hallucinations (all types)	Alcohol in combination can cause extreme sedation, but more often the alcohol causes the medication to be eliminated from the system at a much faster rate, reducing its effectiveness. Nicotine, cocaine, other stimulants also cause medication to be eliminated and make higher doses of medication necessary. Marijuana in daily doses can cause psychosis by itself.	"Jitteriness"	Add medication e.g., artane, cogentin/change to newer medication
	Haloperidal (haldol)	Schizoaffective disorder	Paranoia		Drowsiness	Adjust dose, adjust time of dose, change to newer medication
	Loxapine (loxitane)	Bipolar disorder	Delusions		Inability to relax	Add medication e.g., artane, cogentin/change to newer medication'
	Thioridazine (mellaril)	Major depression with psychosis	Mania (going too fast)		Tight muscles	Add artane or cogentin/change to newer medication
	Thiothixene (navane)	Borderline personality	Thoughts racing		Drooling	Low dose amitriptyline
	Fluphenazine	Paranoid disorder	Thought blocking		Dry mouth	Adjust dose, increase fluids
	Risperidone (risperdal)				Problems with erection	Add medication to counter, change medications
	Quitiepine (seroquel)				Weight gain	Dietary regulation, add newer antiepileptic
	Trifluoperazine				Increase blood sugar	Switch medications
	Chlorpromazine (thorazine)				Effect decreased with cocaine, alcohol, marijuana	Don't use alcohol/other drugs; decrease use, adjust medication upward
	Olanzapine (zyprexa)					
Anti-depressants	Citalopram (cylexa)	Major depression	Sadness	With older antidepressants, mixed with alcohol can be fatal. Newer antidepressants, alcohol reduces effectiveness by causing medication to be eliminated faster and thus reducing the level of medication in the body. Cocaine, etc.	Lethal in combination with alcohol/other depressants	Don't use alcohol/other drugs; switch to newer agent
	Venlafaxine (effexor)	Bipolar illness – depressed phase	Suicidality		Dry mouth	Switch to newer agent
	Amitriptyline (elavil)	Anxiety disorders	Sleep disturbances		Excessive drowsiness	Adjust dose; adjust time of dose
	Desipramine (norpramin)	Pain syndromes	Appetite disturbance		Weight gain	Dietary control; switch to newer agent, add newer antiepileptic medication
	Nortriptyline	Schizophrenia with depression	Anxiousness		Sexual problems	Adjust dose, adjust time of dose, change medication
	Paroxetine (paxil)		Lack of energy		Liver problem	Change medication

Figure 16-12.

Medication family	Example	Illnesses treated	Target symptoms	MEDICATIONS: WHAT THEY DO	Possible problems	Possible remedies
Anti-depressants (continued)	Fluoxetine (prozac)		Unreasonable anger	Do the same thing. In combination with newer medications, may cause psychosis after briefer use.		
	Mirtazapine (remeron)		Impaired concentration			
	Nefazodone					
	Doxepin (sinequan)					
	Imipramine (imipramine)					
	Buproprion (wellbutrin)					
	Sertraline (Zoloft)					
Anti-anxiety medications	Lorazepam (ativan)		Anxiety	Stimulants and these medications each simply counter each other's action. With marijuana, may feel too sleepy, have trouble thinking. In combination with alcohol can be lethal.	Addiction to medication	Avoid use of these medications or use only briefly
	Buspirone (buspar)		Panic attacks		Difficulty remembering	Doesn't happen with Buspar; all others likely
	Clonazepam (klonopin)		Fear of new situations		Excessive drowsiness	Reduce dose or change when given
	Chlordiazepoxide (Librium)	Anxiety disorder	Fear of crowds		Difficulty concentrating	Not as much trouble with Buspar
	Alprazolam (xanax)	Alcohol withdrawal	Generalized feelings of anxiety		Can be lethal in combination with alcohol/other depressants	Don't use alcohol/other drugs or don't use these medications
		Panic disorder			Can give upset stomach	Split dose and give more times per day
Mood stabilizers	Valproic acid (depakote)	Bipolar disorder	Mania (too high)	Alcohol, marijuana, cocaine all causes these medications to be broken down in the system faster so they don't work as well. Have to have increasing amounts of these medications in order for them to work.	Can be dangerous with dehydration	Keep plenty of fluids going especially in hot weather
	Lithium (eskalith, lithobid)	Schizoaffective disorder	Recurring depression		Have to get blood levels checked periodically	Just has to be done
	Carbamazepine (tegretol)	Borderline disorder	Rapid changes in mood			
		Depression when antidepressant alone not enough				

Figure 16-13.

HOW SUBSTANCES OF ABUSE AND MENTAL ILLNESSES INTERACT

Patients know that when they use cocaine they feel better. To pretend otherwise would be silly and diminish the therapist's credibility. They also know the effect wears off and is replaced by a depression that can be quite intense and even life threatening if the person becomes suicidal. Most, however, do not know what the potential problems could be of mixing their medications and the substances they choose to use. Some stop their medications in anticipation of using, fearing a negative interaction.

Figures 16-12 and 16-13 give patients concrete information about how substances of abuse affect medications and recommend how to balance their medications and these same substances. Some would criticize this as giving patients a mixed message. Others would applaud this as giving the patient the knowledge needed to make a truly informed choice.

CASE 16-5

Willie L., 41, had been using cocaine "off and on" for a number of years. Although his usage had substantially decreased over the years, it had not stopped. In the past, he had always discontinued his medications when he went on a cocaine binge. Since his physician had convinced him to stay on his risperidone and valproic acid even if he was using, his rate of hospitalization had plummeted. He was not completely reliable about it, but far better than before. Sometimes he even joked that the doctor had helped him learn how to "get high without getting crazy," and thanked the physician for his thoughtfulness.

Subject Index

Page numbers in italic indicate figures; those followed by a "t" indicate tables.